Learning disabilities: A handbook of integrated care

Edited by
Michael Brown

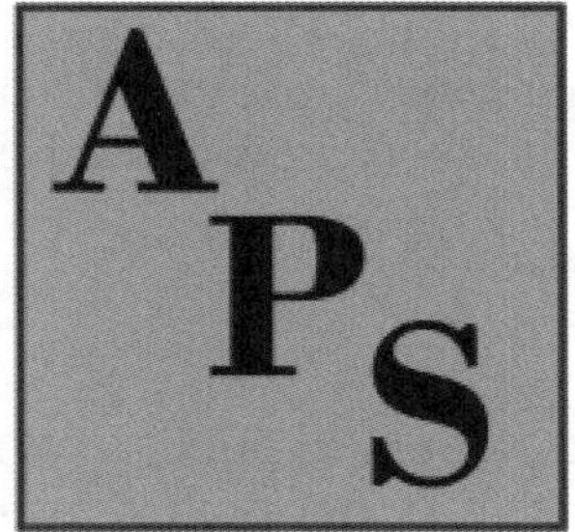

APS Publishing
The Old School, Tollard Royal, Salisbury, Wiltshire, SP5 5PW
www.apspublishing.co.uk

British Library Cataloguing in Publication Data
A catalogue record for this book is available from the British Library

ISBN 1 9038771 9 9

Printed in the United Kingdom by HSW Print, Tonypandy

Contents

Contributors

Mrs Linda Allan *is Senior Nurse and manager of the Primary Care Liaison Team, Greater Glasgow Primary Care NHS Trust*

Mr Michael Brown *is Nurse Consultant with Lothian Primary Care NHS Trust, Edinburgh. He has worked for the Scottish Executive Health Department and NHS Health Scotland on their Learning Disability Health Needs Assessment*

Mrs Lisa Curtice *is the Director of the Scottish Consortium for Learning Disability which is based in Glasgow*

Dr Fergus Douds *is Consultant Psychiatrist, and currently works for the Intellectual Disability Dual Diagnosis Service, Capital and Coast District Health Board, Wellington, New Zealand*

Dr Ros Lyall *is Consultant Psychiatrist and Clinical Director for learning disability services, Lothian Primary Care NHS Trust, Edinburgh*

Mrs Juliet MacArthur *is Senior Nurse: Research, Lothian University Hospitals NHS Trust, Western General Hospital, Edinburgh*

Dr Tommy MacKay *is a Psychologist, Psychology Consultancy Services, Ardoch House, Cardross, Dumbartonshire G82 5E*

Professor Roy McConkey *is Professor of Learning Disability, University of Ulster and Eastern Health & Social Services Board, Northern Ireland*

Mr David Marshall *is a Lecturer, Department of Nursing Studies, Queens University, Northern Ireland*

Dr Craig Melville *is Senior Lecturer, Section of Psychological Medicine, University of Glasgow and Honorary Consultant Psychiatrist, Greater Glasgow Primary Care NHS Trust*

Mr Gordon Moore *is Principal Nurse with Down Lisburn Health and Social Care Trust, Northern Ireland*

Professor Jillian Morrison *is Professor of General Practice at the University of Glasgow and is a practising General Practitioner*

Dr Walter Muir *is Reader in the Psychiatry of Learning Disability, School of Molecular and Clinical Medicine, College of Medicine and Veterinary Medicine, University of Edinburgh, and Honorary Consultant Psychiatrist, Lothian Primary Care NHS Trust*

Dr Douglas Paterson *is Specialist Registrar in the Psychiatry of Learning Disability, West of Scotland Higher Specialist Training Scheme*

Mrs Janette Rennie *is a Physiotherapist who has worked extensively with people with learning disabilities. She has recently retired from clinical practice and continues to have an interest in the care and support of people with learning disabilities*

Dr Elita Smiley *is Specialist Registrar in the Psychiatry of Learning Disability, West of Scotland Higher Specialist Training Scheme*

Mrs Jenny Whinnett *is the mother of Craig, a young man with learning disabilities, and works for PAMIS, an organisation that offers support to the family carers of people with profound and multiple learning disabilities*

Dr Margaret Whoriskey *is Disability Advisor, NHS Quality Improvement Scotland, Edinburgh*

Foreword

The landscape of Learning Disability is constantly changing. New horizons emerge that present exciting challenges to people with learning disabilities and truly improve their quality of life. To achieve these life opportunities and enhanced personal goals skilled staff from a variety of disciplines will be required to facilitate, guide and support. This in itself not only presents challenges to people with learning disabilities, but to the staff working with them. In the case of the latter, much reflection on role definition and professional practice may be required. The context for service delivery could alter as an outcome of this changing landscape.

Reflective practice is key for all staff working with people with learning disabilities in the twenty-first century. As such, the recognition of a whole range of professional disciplines as evidence-based is crucial. The role of research that is practitioner-based can make a major contribution to this process. Collaborative research involving professionals from a variety of backgrounds could significantly move forward integrated service delivery, as it would stem from a shared agenda with common goals, and focussed outcomes (Forbes, 2003). Some professional groups are further along that path than others, but it is a point that all must reach if we are to achieve the integrated care advocated by this book. Indeed, there is a strong case for abandoning terminology, such as multi-disciplinary, multi-professional or even interdisciplinary, and look towards a transdisciplinary model of service delivery. Our adherence to the structures of our various professional disciplines creates boundaries. These boundaries are unhelpful to people with learning disabilities and their families who may need to interact with a range of professionals. We need to evolve models of practice that can transcend these disciplinary boundaries, leading to a unified model of service delivery. Such approaches would be truly integrated and certainly person-centred.

For integration and inclusion to be successful, we need to be mindful of the population of people with learning disabilities who we are seeking to serve and support. This is a changing population. For example, the prevalence of children and adults with autistic spectrum disorders is subject to constant revision, (as McKay, *Chapter 10*, points out).

With technological progress and developments in medical practice, the survival rates of neonates are increasing (Emsley *et al*, 1998). A significant proportion of these children will be born with major disabilities and will require the lifelong support of professional services (Carpenter, 1999). Professionals will need to plan ahead and, with families, explore new ways of intervening in order to improve the quality of life (Whoriskey, *Chapter 4*) for the next generation, and to ensure that inclusion is more than an aspiration; rather it is a reality.

Curtice (*Chapter 3*) poses some human rights and equality issues in relation to inclusion. In the 'Valuing People' White Paper the whole thrust of inclusion is underscored by rights, independence and choice (DoH, 2001). This major policy acknowledges that for the inclusion of people with learning disabilities to be successful, there are still many barriers in society to be broken down. However, we need to cling to our high expectations of people with learning disabilities, celebrating their achievements and developing opportunities for them to interact widely with their communities. This will best be achieved by joined-up services working in true collaboration in supporting the lives of the people they serve. This is a resounding message of this book.

A deep and meaningful understanding of inclusion is critical if services are to achieve this goal. Over time, Lewis (1995) suggests integration became a too narrowly interpreted concept. It had failed to align itself to the more socially-permeated concept of normalisation and thus many professionals sought a concept that was more holistic in its outlook. The concept of inclusion emerged and advocated the belief that people with learning disabilities belong in the mainstream of society.

The challenge of this approach has initially been kindled in the context of schools (Carpenter and Shevlin, 2003). A move is afoot to look at inclusive schools as organisations capable of accepting diversity, with strategies to meet a range of individual needs. This approach has been mirrored across service development in other major disciplines, as articulated in this book. In the spirit of Mittler's (2000) views on inclusive education, it is possible to look at the wider social context and realise that meaningful inclusion (as a quality of life process for the person with learning disabilities) is not just about being placed in mainstream services. It is about changing society as a whole to make it more responsive to the needs of all people; and within services it is about helping all professionals to accept their responsibility to deliver services to all, regardless of a person's disability.

Some would interpret this stance as advocating the abolition of specialist learning disability services. This is not so. Inclusion will only be successful where there are a range of differentiated services capable of meeting a range of individual needs, but within the context of an integrated service. Fergus Douds (*Chapter 11*) decries the artificial dichotomy between 'health' and 'social care' (and I would add 'education'). He goes on to state:

> *"Effective joint working should reduce duplication of services and lead to more efficient provision. It should also result in agencies taking collective responsibility for problems. Ultimately, joined-up planning and working by professionals is necessary, if integrated community services are to be provided, drawing on the strengths of professionals from a range of backgrounds".*
>
> (p233)

Service development for people with learning disabilities requires a lifespan approach (Cuskelly *et al*, 2002), mobilising communities, empowering families and ensuring that a policy framework is in place that can facilitate not only good service provision, but can deliver the goals, aspirations and dreams of people with learning disabilities.

Workforce development is crucial as a focus throughout. One of the key recommendations of the Inquiry into Meeting the Mental Health Needs of Young People with Learning

Disabilities (FPLD, 2002) was the development of shared learning across professional groups at induction, in-service, undergraduate and postgraduate levels. In various forms and tiers of training, we could thus ensure that professionals at generalist and specialist levels were equipped with sound knowledge and skills in relation to people with learning disabilities, set in a framework of positive attitudes and service entitlement. This book will go a long way to enable a range of professional groups to achieve their goals. Its focus on integrated care and service delivery is timely and will encourage critical reflection upon service structures and styles of service delivery, as befits the lives of people with learning disabilities in this twenty-first century.

September 2003

Barry Carpenter OBE
Chief Executive, Sunfield
Honorary Professor
University of Northumbria

References

Carpenter B, Shevlin M (2003) Creating an inclusive curriculum. In: Walsh PN, Gash H, eds. *Lives and Times: People with Intellectual Disabilities—A Lifecourse Approach*. Wordwell, Dublin, Ireland

Carpenter B (1999) Perspective. *Infants Young Children* **12**(1): 4–10

Cuskelly M, Jobling A, Buckley S, eds (2002) *Down Syndrome Across the Lifespan*. Whurr Publications, London

Department of Health (2001) *Valuing People: A New Strategy for the 21st Century*. The Stationery Office, London

Emsley H, Wardle S, Sims D, Chiswick M, D'Souza S (1998) Increased services and deteriorating developmental outcomes in 23–25 week old gestation infants in 1990–94 compared with 1984–89. *Arch Dis Childhood* **78**(2): 113–29

Forbes J (2003) Grappling with collaboration: would opening up the research 'base' help? *Br J Spec Educ* **30**(3): 150–55

Foundation for People with Learning Disabilities (2002) *Count Us In*. The report of the Committee of Inquiry into Meeting the Mental Health Needs of Young People with Learning Disabilities. Mental Health Foundation, London

Lewis A (1995) *Children's Understanding of Disability*. Routledge, London
Mittler P (2000) *Working Towards Inclusive Education: Social Contexts*. David Fulton, London

Introduction

Learning Disabilities: A handbook of integrated care brings together some of the important issues that impact on the care and support of people with learning disabilities in the twenty-first century. The main themes that run throughout are the changes that have taken place and brought people with learning disabilities to the point where they are articulating their needs and speaking for themselves—they are demanding to be visible and heard.

Integration, and the journey towards this, is a key theme, as is the support needs of people with learning disabilities and others with the most challenging needs, such as those with autism and mental ill-health. The book picks up on issues that need to be considered in order for inclusion and integration to take place for a group of people who have, historically, not been considered. The chapter contributors are all experts in their area and have extensive experience in working with people with learning disabilities, and their carers.

The book is aimed at a wide audience who have an interest in people with learning disabilities. It is relevant to those involved in the care and support of people with learning disabilities who wish to update their knowledge, and for those who have already undertaken study that includes a focus on people with learning disabilities. The audience will also include students from a range of study programmes in health and social care—medical, nursing, therapists and professions allied to health, social work, and education, as well as those in the voluntary sector. It will also be of interest and relevant to family carers who are concerned with the care and support of their loved ones. This book is very relevant to people who think that people with learning disabilities are 'none of their business'.

The key areas covered in *Learning Disabilities: A Handbook of Integrated Care* are:

• Policy and Practice	• Addressing inequalities
• Listening to and involving people with learning disabilities	• Quality and monitoring
• Ethics and genetics	• Legislation and the law
• A carer's perspective	• Health surveillance and improvement
• Promoting health and integration	• Autism
• Mental well-being	• Older people with learning disabilities

The book is divided in to two sections:

The first chapter by ***Michael Brown and Jeanette Rennie*** opens with the policy and legislation that has impacted on the lives of people with learning disabilities. It highlights the developments that have taken place internationally and concludes with recent policy developments.

Michael Brown and Douglas Paterson consider the health inequalities experienced by people with learning disabilities, and models of health improvement that seek to address such inequalities, and promote social inclusion and integration.

Lisa Curtice draws on models and theories of social disability and contrasts these with the traditional medical model, outlining how people with learning disabilities are being supported in their efforts to have their voice heard and, as a result, take control of their lives.

Margaret Whoriskey explores the important issue of quality and monitoring of care for some of the most vulnerable people within our society, describing examples of where this occurs and how people with learning disabilities can be included.

Walter Muir examines the contentious issue of genetics and the impact of developments from an ethical perspective in a historical and contemporary context.

Ros Lyall looks at the legal and legislative contexts and considers, specifically, the challenges surrounding the capacity to give consent. She goes on to discuss the rights of people with learning disabilities under The Human Rights Act.

The second part goes on to look at the challenges presented when working towards integration of people with learning disabilities, who are among some of the most disadvantaged and excluded within societies—people with learning disabilities who have autism, mental ill health, are offenders, and older people with learning disabilities.

Jennie Whinette writes about her son, Craig, a young man with profound and multiple learning disabilities, and draws on her experience, as his mother, to outline the real life experience.

David Marshall, Gordon Moore, and Roy McConkey outline a research project involving people with learning disabilities that looked at a wide range of needs—unidentified and unmet—and goes on to explore the responses required to address them.

Craig Melville, Jillian Morrison, Linda Allan and Juliet MacArthur explore the issues around the greater health needs of people with learning disabilities, and give practical examples from practice in primary care and general hospital services that seek to ensure appropriate access and support is available.

Tommy McKay looks at the issue of autistic spectrum disorder and Asperger's Syndrome—and the relatively recent recognition of the needs of this group—and the challenges involved in their inclusion and support.

Fergus Douds explores issues surrounding mental well being of people with learning disabilities and the common areas of mental ill health. He goes on to explore the challenges of working with people with learning disabilities who have forensic needs, and how services can work to include them and take account of their needs.

Elita Smilie concludes with the chapter about older people with learning disabilities, considers their needs as they age and the particular issues that need to be looked at in order to ensure that these needs are met. This is an important topic, as there is limited experience of the increasing number of older people with learning disabilities and how they age.

1
From policy to practice

Michael Brown and Jeanette Rennie

This chapter is written under sub headings, which explore the historical development of policy and legislation that have impacted on the lives of people with learning disabilities. It identifies key changes that have occurred up to the current day, which have resulted in the gradual change in attitudes, leading to a concept of integration and inclusion. It is important to consider the policy developments within their historical context and time, and recognise how thinking has changed and evolved. Tables are used to show development of terminology and major changes that have taken place.

Integrated and inclusive care for people with learning disabilities, intellectual disabilities, or mental retardation conjures up and implies different things to different people. The term used differs according to geography across continents; however, the needs are by and large the same the world over. What differs is the range of policy approaches and initiatives that have been developed, across the Western world, in an attempt to provide what has been considered, historically, to be appropriate care and support. The World Health Organization continues to uses the term 'mental retardation', with 'intellectual disability' now more frequently used. 'Mental handicap' is the term that continues to be used in many developing countries. For the purposes of this book, the term *learning disability* will be used throughout.

To some, integrated and inclusive care means people with learning disabilities living visibly and included in their community and, to others, the idea of collaborative working between professions or integration of service providers to provide care and support in mainstream services. To many it will mean a combination of all of these.

Since a Danish Act of Parliament in 1959 stated that, '*Whatever facilities are open to all other citizens must, in principle, also be available to the mentally retarded*', there has been a gradual, if uneven, worldwide move to recognise and work towards the integration of people with learning disabilities into the community. A statutory report of midwives referred to, what was to become known as, 'community care' in 1955. A significant step forward was made when Bank Mikkelsen and Bengt Nirje brought the concept of normalisation fully into view of all those working with people with learning disabilities in 1969, when Nirje published, 'The normalisation principle and its human management implications'. The changes and developments in policy, attitude, and thinking have been gradual and, in the past, not based around the needs and aspirations of people with learning disabilities.

Who are people with learning disabilities?

It is important to recognise that people with learning disabilities, their families and carers have brought about the biggest and most significant changes that have impacted upon the care and support of people with learning disabilities. In the UK, in 1995, a ground swell of opinion from people who were at that time referred to as "mentally handicapped " their families and those who worked with them, brought about a change in terminology from *mental handicap* to *learning disability*. This term has now been integrated into every day language and has been adopted by government in publications, such as, *The Health of the Nation: A Strategy for People with learning Disabilities*, part of the wider study *The Health of the Nation* (England and Wales) and later again in the English Department of Health strategy *Valuing People: A New Strategy for Learning Disability for the 21st Century* (2001). In Scotland, the Scottish Executive published *The Same as You? A review of services for people with learning disabilities in 2000.* Within these strategies, a learning disability was said to exist when there is:

- A significantly reduced ability to understand new or complex information, to learn new skills (impaired intelligence); with
- A reduced ability to cope independently (impaired social functioning);
- Which started before adulthood, with a lasting effect on development.

Professionals concerned with the care and support of people with learning disabilities, such as the medical profession, have developed definitions of learning disability that are detailed in ICD-10, AAMR or DSM-IV.

However, the general public continue to associate 'learning' solely with education and elsewhere in the world other terminology reflects this understanding. For example in the United States the term learning disability was introduced in 1962 to mean:

> *'A disorder in one or more of the basic psychological processes involved in the understanding or in using language, spoken or written, which may manifest itself in an incomplete ability to listen, think, speak, read, write or spell, or to do mathematical calculations'*...it includes: *'perceptual handicaps, dyslexia, developmental aphasia, brain injury, mid brain dysfunction.'*

Development of terminology in relation to provision of care

The range of terminology, adopted over the years, needs to be read in context with the life and times in which it was used. It is a marker of the way in which people with learning disabilities were seen within the society they lived. What is now regarded as condescending was frequently caring and progressive, and many philanthropists, educationalists, health professionals, and sociologists have contributed to political decision-making that influenced and impacted upon the ways in which people with learning disabilities were cared for. Before the introduction of modern medicines, only those who would now be regarded as having mild to moderate learning disability would have survived beyond infancy.

Shakespeare's plays indicate that, until the early 1600s, people with learning disabilities were an accepted and, in some cases, revered part of the community, as people 'possessed' or with 'second sight', who influenced everyday occurrences and major battles. This said, Morris (1969), Trent (1994), and Scherenberger (1987) state that some might also be locked up and ill-treated. This ill treatment may have been linked to various 'tests', which were devised to verify 'fools', both to protect them and to gain their property rights. Categories devised by Wilbur in the late 1890s illustrated the expectations for people with, even what were considered as, the most severe learning disabilities. Such terms, when viewed within the current social context, appear cruel and abhorrent.

- '**simulative idiots**: could be prepared for ordinary duties and enjoyments of humanity
- **higher grade idiots**: would attend common schools to be qualified for civil usefulness and social happiness
- **lower-grade idiots**: could become decent in their habits, educated in simple occupations, capable of self-support under judicious management in their own families, or in public industrial institutions for adult idiots.
- **incurables**: aim to achieve some education'.

(Trent, 1994)

Table 1:1 Examples of key dates in the development of terminology and definitions

Year	Country	Terminology/Definition
Late 1890	UK	Feeble-minded, imbecile, idiot
1913	UK	Moral imbecile, feeble-minded, imbecile, idiot
1921	US (AAMR)	American Association on Mental Retardation (AAMR) published 'Manual on Terminology and Classification in Mental Retardation
1959	UK	Legal terminology England and Wales: subnormal, severe subnormal (also used 'mental handicap' and 'severe mental handicap'). Scotland: mental deficiency, severe mental deficiency
1968	WHO	Mental retardation: mild, moderate, severe, profound
1973	US (AAMR)	Mental retardation refers to significantly sub average, general intellectual functioning, existing concurrently with deficits in adaptive behaviour and manifested during the developmental period (Grossman, 1973)
1978	UK	Education terminology England and Wales: learning difficulties replaced educationally subnormal (moderate and severe)
1980	WHO	International Classification of Impairments, Disabilities and Handicaps; Mental retardation—all people with IQ of <70
1981	UK	Education terminology one category: learning difficulty
1983	UK (England and Wales)	'**Mental impairment**: a state of arrested or incomplete development of mind, which includes a significant impairment of intelligence and social functioning, and is associated with abnormally aggressive or seriously irresponsible conduct on the part of the person concerned' (Mental Health Act, 1983)
1983	UK (Scotland)	Mental handicap replaced mental deficiency, but had the same general meaning (Mental Health (Scotland) Act, 1983)

Year	Country	Terminology/Definition
1992	WHO and US (AAMR)	'International Classification of Impairments, Disabilities and Handicaps [ICD 10]'. Mental retardation: accepted terminology, but definition updated
1994	US (APA)	American Psychiatric Association DSM-IV; Mental retardation: accepted terminology
1995	UK	Learning disability: accepted terminology (DoH, 1995). Medically, used in conjunction with more specific definition

Key dates in the development of terminology and definitions abridged from Rennie (2001)

What predated integrated care?

Prior to the industrial revolution, people who were well-known locally were an accepted part of everyday life, although the introduction of Vagrancy Acts in the UK in 1713 reflected a fear that unknown people with learning disabilities might be dangerous. In France during the early nineteenth century, positive treatment and teaching were introduced by Itard (Lane, 1977), Pinel (Trent, 1994) and Seguin (Kanner, 1964). This was something that had never been considered before. Itard began to use baths for training purposes for mental defectives, although not as an attempt to improve physical abilities, despite them being used for such purposes with the general population in Spas throughout Europe.

Institutions

A dichotomy of care and fear developed during the 19th century, with the establishment of institutions to promote education and care by philanthropic reformers, such as Dr and Mrs Brodie, who founded the Edinburgh Idiot Asylum in 1855, later to become The Royal Scottish National Institute for Mental Defectives (Henderson, 1964). At the same time, however, the idea that low intellectual ability was an entirely inherited factor, 'the degeneration theory', was proposed. The fear of hereditary transmission grew, as people were categorised by tests that took no account of environmental and social conditions, or physical disabilities.

The fear of a great expansion in the numbers of 'mental defectives' became so great that Tredgold's article in the Eugenics review (1909), 'The Feebleminded: a social danger', is thought to have influenced the decision to add a statutory instrument to the Mental Deficiency Act of 1913. This separated 'mentally deficient' people from the general population and from the opposite sex. However, it was not until 1927 that differences were officially acknowledged and separate institutions were introduced for people with mental illness and those with mental handicap.

By 1936, the institutions were beginning to be known as colonies, and were sited in rural areas for the safety of their residents. Attitudes did not remain static, however, and further questions arose for staff of these colonies in ensuring the most appropriate treatment and management for each category of resident. It began to be accepted that the 'lower grades' needed custodial lifetime care, but the most 'able' residents were trained sufficiently to work in the community (Loudon, 1992).

The UK 1948 Health Service Act insisted that senior doctors working in 'subnormality hospitals' were appropriately qualified. It also gave responsibility to local authorities to find accommodation for anyone needing care and attention, in temporary establishments if necessary. This raised the number of residents and the number of hospitals and colonies considerably. Again, a dichotomy occurred where the residents were being accommodated safely in a large rural establishment, but away from urban areas where medical staff, nurses and therapists trained, worked, and found professional support from other colleagues. The hospitals became isolated communities that were frequently the main source of employment for local villages.

Table 1:2 Examples of key developments world wide prior to the movement towards integrated care

Year	Country	
1713–1714	UK	Vagrancy Acts: apprehension of those who might be dangerous
1774	UK	Madhouses Act: provision of minimum standards of care and for the control of private madhouses
1808	UK	Country Asylums Acts: public asylums in England replaced private madhouses
1839	Switzerland	Guggenbuhl established a 'colony' on the Abendberg
1820–1860	USA	The Depression, Civil War and ideas from Europe and Britain led to 'indoor relief' replacing 'outdoor relief', residential asylums for training feeble-minded adults and idiots replacing schools for feeble-minded children and medically trained superintendents replacing head teachers
1908	UK	Report of Royal Commission on Care and Control of the Feeble-minded
1913	UK	Mental Deficiency Act: People with mental deficiency dealt with as a specific group. Segregation introduced. Mental defectives classified
1927	UK	Mental Deficiency Act: Creation of separate institutions for the mentally ill and mentally handicapped
1948	UK	The National Health Service Act (as amended) standardised mental subnormality hospitals in line with general hospitals
1958	USA	Anthony Dexter conceived a 'social system concept'
1959	UK	Mental Health Act repealed all previous legislation. Voluntary admission to hospital emphasised. Civil rights of patients recognised, including access to a Health Service Commissioner

World-wide developments prior to the movement towards integrated care; (compiled from Morris, 1969; Scheerenberger, 1987; Trent, 1994; and abridged from Rennie, 2001)

Beginning to look outwards

The Royal Commission on the Law Relating to Mental Illness and Mental Deficiency (1957) and the Mental Health Act (1959) were the UK government's response to publication of injustices done to people classified as 'moral defectives', who had been sent to institutions for life, following incidents relating to adolescent aggression or promiscuity. This made many members of the general public aware of the anomaly, which arose partly from trying to ensure that 'mentally defective' people who had committed more serious offences were held in custody in a hospital rather than a gaol. These developments should be considered within their historical context. In their day, they were viewed as forward thinking, just as developments in the twenty-first century are seen today. How will the recent policy and practice developments be seen in fifty years? The idea of sanctuary, in the truest sense, led to the development of colonies for people with learning disabilities in the nineteenth century, where there was a focus on training and work, often in areas such as farming.

The 1959 Mental Health Act promoted a change in attitude and towards the subject of 'mental handicap' that, in turn, began to encourage greater voluntary involvement and recognition of people with learning disabilities by the general public.

Expanding services within the hospitals

Despite the fact that the proposal for a reduction in the numbers of people living in mental hospitals was first recommended by the Minister of Health in 1961, numbers continued to rise until the early 1970s (Brown ,1992). The idea was partly an attempt to save money and partly to improve conditions for the residents and remove the stigma surrounding them. (Scrivens, 1986).

Gradually, it became accepted that people with learning disabilities were not 'ill' and did not require hospitals to be their homes. The need for on-going nursing and health care should be provided for those who require it in a community setting. (Scheerenberger, 1987) People with learning disabilities, who also had physical disabilities, required the type of active treatment being made available to children with physical disabilities and average intelligence (Bobath and Bobath, 1975; Hari and Akos, 1988). Without such important provision, there was a possibility that children and adults with additional physical disabilities would develop deformities that would inhibit their ability to leave hospital.

The terminology of subnormal, mental deficiency and mental retardation continued to create an attitude of stigma towards both hospital residents and the professional staff who worked with them. They were also terms that were indicative of repressive conditions found in some hospitals at that time. This said, it is important to remember that, overall, very few people with learning disabilities were ever in the long-stay hospitals. The majority have always lived in the community, with family carers providing care and support, often with limited help. The deteriorating conditions that became apparent in the long-stay hospitals led to many family carers seeing them as a very poor last resort.

Despite the overcrowding that began to occur within the long-stay hospitals, there were attempts to provide education, therapy, and treatment for those with the greatest need. For example, remedial gymnasts began to hear about learning disability during their training and, in conjunction with nursing staff, organised and developed sporting activities for more physically able residents. Frequently, occupational therapists had worked initially in psychiatric hospitals, while speech and physiotherapists had seen the need for their specific therapy from the perspective of paediatrics or neurology. For example, physiotherapists who had worked with Karel and Berta Bobath when they introduced their method of working with children with cerebral palsy (Bobath and Bobath, 1975; Mayston, 2002) continued to work with children, and then adults, in Harpebury Hospital. In Edinburgh, one occupational therapist transferred from a psychiatric hospital, speech therapists were initially seconded from The Scottish Council for Spastics (now Capability Scotland), and the physiotherapist had previously worked with physically and mentally handicapped children in Norway.

In some hospitals, new professions set up their own departments in isolation from each other and from the wards. In others, the opposite was true, as therapists understood that they could not bring the greatest benefit to the residents without help and support, whether this was in their own department, on the wards, or outside the hospital. In such hospitals, nursing staff also realised that this was a different and potentially useful intervention. Paediatric and orthopaedic consultants began to establish clinics in addition to those already run by psychiatrists.

The start of community integration—a visit to an airport

- **People involved:**

Young adults, aged fourteen to sixteen years with moderate to severe learning disabilities, none fully independent. Conditions included: a chromosomal abnormality involving contractures, and subsequent sore areas at knees and elbows, Down's syndrome and delayed speech maturation, and cerebral palsy with hemiplegia, poor lip closure and poor swallowing.

- **Staff involved:**

Speech therapist, physiotherapist, and occupational therapist with occasional assistance from a social worker from a local voluntary funded organisation. Hospital ward staff ensured that patients were dressed appropriately and brought them to the physiotherapy department.

- Aims

  Therapeutic and medical:
  - To improve general mobility
  - To improve lower limb range of movement
  - To improve lip closure and swallowing
  - To improve communication skills
  - To improve hand skills.

  Social
  - To visit a place of interest
  - To be among people other than hospital residents

- To have fun.

A visit to the local small airport

- Patients encouraged to get themselves in and out of the car with minimal assistance
- Walk into and around the airport including up and down stairs to the viewing gallery
- Patients encouraged to select their own cold drink and cake or biscuit in the café, and
- Patients encouraged to use toilet facilities.

This gradual and often patchy progress continued in collaboration between private, charitably run facilities and health service hospitals into the 1970s. For example, in Edinburgh hospitals, 'patients' married, returned briefly to their long stay hospital and then moved into flats supported by community services. Throughout the UK, children with a learning disability were beginning to be supported in integrated education, as attitudes towards inclusion developed.

The journeys towards integration and inclusion

Table 1:3 First steps towards 'integration'

Year	Country	
1959	Denmark	The government passed 'An Act concerning Care of the Mentally Retarded and other Exceptionally Retarded Persons'
1961	USA	President Kennedy appointed a President's Panel on mental retardation
1961	UK	Minister of Health proposed start of 'running down' mental hospitals
1969	USA	Concept of Normalisation introduced by Bank Mikkelsen and Bengt Nirje
Early **1970s**	Canada	Responsibility for people with mental handicap transferred from health to social welfare and educational ministries
1970s	Australia	Several states acted upon reports recommending mentally handicapped people transfer to the community

Year	Country	
1971	UN	Declaration on the Rights of Mentally Retarded Persons
1971	UK	'Better Services for the Mentally Handicapped'
1971	USA	International League of Societies for the Mentally Handicapped endorsed philosophy of normalisation
1975	UK	The National Development Group and National Development for the Mentally Handicapped established
1975	UN	Declaration of the Rights of Disabled People
1978	UK	'Helping Mentally Handicapped People in Hospital'
1978	UK	Warnock Committee Report on special educational needs
1979	UK	Jay Report. Policy based on principles of normalisation. Special help would be required from their communities and the professional services. Advocacy recommended. 'A Better Life' (Scotland). Concept of community care endorsed; gradual progress recommended.
1980	WHO	'International Classification of Impairments, Disabilities and Handicaps'
1980	UK	SHAPE (Scottish Health Authorities Priorities for the Eighties)
1981	UK	Education Act for Children with Special Education Needs and Education (Scotland) Act. Education should be fitted to the child's requirements as far as possible. Statement of needs and needs assessments proposed
1983	UK	The All Wales Strategy
1983	UK	Mental Health Act
1984	UK	The Mental Health (Scotland) Act
1986	UK	The Disabled Persons Act (Tom Clarke Act). Right to representation, assessment, information, consultation. Carers right to ask for assessment of disabled person's needs and have carer's ability to care taken into account
1987	USA	The Developmental Disabilities Assistance and Bill of Rights Amendments include persons with mental retardation

Year	Country	
1987	UK	Mental Handicap: Progress, Problems and Priorities: A Review of Mental Handicap Services in England since the 1971 White Paper
1988	UK	Community Care: Agenda for Action (Griffiths Report)
1988	UK	SHARPEN (Scottish Health Authorities Review of Priorities for the Eighties and Nineties)
1989	UK	White Paper 'Caring for People: community Care in the Next Decade and Beyond'
1990	UK	NHS and Community Care Act. Confirmed proposals in 1989 White Paper
1990	Sweden	Recommended that all institutions close
1995	UK	'The Health of the Nation' including 'A Strategy for People with Learning Disabilities and Their Carers'
1998	UK	'Signposts for Success'
1999	UK	The Health Act
2001	Scotland	The Same as You?
2002	England	Valuing People

Adapted and abridged from Rennie 2001

The 1970s –support for community integration

The 1970s saw the development if ideas and policy, aimed at the inclusion of people with learning disabilities from long-stay hospitals into the community. In 1971, the government published 'Better service for the mentally handicapped'. Considerable change and developments have taken place over the past three decades. There has been a move towards enabling people with learning disabilities to lead ordinary and inclusive lives in the community. There has been a policy to close long-stay hospitals and develop alternative social models of support within the community. These developments were given added stimulus by The National Development Team (NDT), which was established to facilitate progress from hospitals to the community. This was helped by realignment of funding from central government, increased involvement of social services departments, and the effect of The Warnock Report (1978) on special educational needs. A range of international and national policy statements began to shape the thinking about the care and support required by people with learning

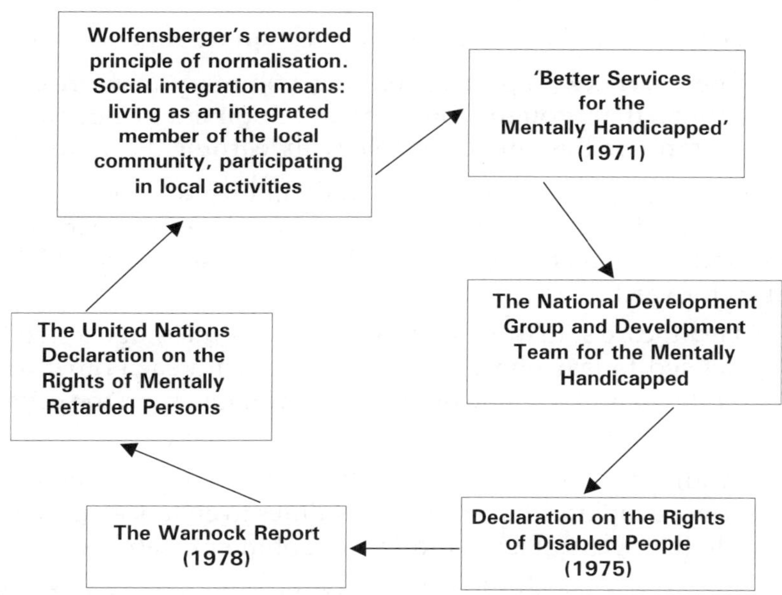

Moves towards community integration in the 1970s

disabilities.

The United Nations Declaration on the Rights of Mentally Retarded Persons coincided with the publication of 'Better Services for the Mentally Handicapped' in the United Kingdom. . The United Nations Declaration on the Rights of Disabled People (1975) stated that :

> *'Whatever the origin, nature and seriousness of their handicaps and disabilities, they have the same fundamental rights of their*

> *fellow citizens of the same age, which implies first and foremost the right to enjoy a decent life, as normal and as full as possible.'*

Many of the developments that were taking place during the 1970s began at 'grass roots' level where there was a new impetus led by:

- An increasing awareness among families of the needs of their family member
- A growth in the development of voluntary organisations
- The Warnock Report generating voluntary and pressure groups that brought about the development of campaigns to improve the care for people with learning disabilities.

There were, however, increasing recognition and concerns that significant obstacles needed to be overcome before true integration and inclusion for people with learning disabilities could be taken forward:

- Healthcare staff, social services and voluntary agency staff, needed to learn how to work closely with each other and understand the value of the skills available from the different groups
- Additional support from health services was required by some people with learning disabilities to enhance quality of life that was not a re-enforcement of their disability
- Increasing recognition that making choices is essential to individual social development
- The valuable skills of health professionals needed to be translated in to the community, where the majority of people with learning disabilities lived
- Some hospital staff were reluctant and wary of moving into the community (Allan *et al*, 1990).

The 1980s and 1990s: An uneven progress

As with any change resulting from the discovery of mistakes that have been made, there was a tendency to move rapidly in the opposite direction. Such recognition was the rapid move towards the closure of long-stay hospitals in England, and a more gradual approach in Scotland, Wales and Northern Ireland. The numbers of people with learning disabilities living in hospitals began to fall dramatically. The 'All Wales Strategy' was published 1983 and brought with it an emphasis on the principles of normalisation. The closure of long-stay hospitals brought a new focus on the health needs of people with learning disabilities, and questions were asked about the generic health care available. There was a gradual recognition that many of the health needs of people with learning disabilities were not being effectively addressed, and this lack of recognition also applied to many other areas, i.e.employment. Policy that began to emerge encompassed the following:

- O'Brien's five essential qualities for life: community presence, choice, competence, respect and community participation (Tyne and O'Brien, 1981)
- Wolfensberger's redefinition of normalisation as Social Role Valorisation (SRV): 'The enablement, establishment, enhancement, maintenance, and/or defence of valued social roles for people—particularly for those at value risk—by using, as much as possible, culturally valued means' (Wolfensberger and Thomas, 1983)
- Kristiansen and Ness (1987) additional accomplishments for quality of life: expression of individuality and experience of continuity in one's own life.

The publication of 'Caring for People' (Department of Health, 1989) transferred assessment of need from health to social services, and increased the responsibility of care expected of families and the voluntary services.

Wolfensberger's further reworded definition of 'normalisation' in 1992, which differentiated between valuing a person for him/herself, and ensuring that the person fulfilled a valued role, gave impetus to a number of community projects.

In the early 1990s, health care professionals expressed concern about the facilities that would be available for the management and treatment of those with the most severe and profound learning disabilities moving from long stay hospitals. It became evident that the infrastructures required within the community had not been developed to support people with such complex needs, and that capital continued to be tied up in hospital provision (Turner *et al*, 1995). Slower progress of hospital closure was made in Scotland and many of the lessons learned were written into 'Recommendations of the future of Mental Handicap Hospitals' (Loudon, 1992).

A positive step forward occurred with the publication of 'The Health of the Nation' by the Department of Health in 1995. The term 'learning disability' was recognised and an accompanying publication, 'The Health of the Nation: A Strategy for People with Learning Disabilities' (Department of Health, 1992) was written, specifically, to focus on the needs of the group. It was also the first time the range of health needs that could affect people with learning disabilities was clearly stated in a national document. These included:

- Obesity
- Poor cardiovascular fitness
- Behavioural problems
- Psychiatric problems
- Orthopaedic problems
- Mobility problems.

This implicitly explained the need for wide-ranging professional involvement, among people with learning disabilities, to ensure that they were able to make the most of opportunities becoming available in the community. It also facilitated the use of multi-professional community learning disability teams, and enabled the individual health profession groups to clarify their specific work to their peers in other areas of the health service.

In the late 1990s, 'Signposts for Success' was published. The report made specific recommendations for Community Learning Disability Health Services:

- Provision of co-ordinated support, advice and training for people with learning disabilities their families and carers

- Provision of therapeutic services
- Assistance with good health care promotion and practice
- Close working with other agencies and facilitating access to general health services.

The following case studies are examples of how these aims have been at least partially met.

Case study one: Keeping yourself health

Accessible information

- A series about specific health needs, such as testicular self-examination, breast examination and dental care that were prepared for everyday use by people with learning disabilities, family carers and health professionals, such as primary care teams and community learning disability nurses.

Leaflets

- Produced by FAIR (Family and Information Resource and Advice for People with Learning Disabilities) in collaboration with Lothian Primary Care NHS Trust, Learning Disability Team in Edinburgh.

Funded

- By the Health Education Board of Scotland.

Case study two: Working in partnership with mainstream services

Community learning disability nurses working as an integral part of a homeless people's health team with:

- General practitioners
- Practice nurse
- Mental health nurses
- District nurses.

Additional services provided by the practice:

- General health care
- Bathing
- Changes of clothes.

Working collaboratively within the same building as:

- Housing
- Social work.

Case study three: co-ordinated work between clinics and health trusts

The client

A woman, aged 43 years at the time of first referral. She had mild learning disabilities and challenging behaviour. Prior to the initial episode, she had joined a once weekly physiotherapy-led Scottish country dance session. This aimed to improve general levels of fitness and co-ordination, through a normal Scottish activity.

Initial episode

- Moderate damage to an Achilles tendon during a sporting activity
- Referred to the community learning disability team (CLDT) physiotherapist by a community physiotherapist after five treatment sessions at the local medical practice
- Treated individually once weekly and returned to country dancing.

Second episode

- Fractured first metacarpal during handball
- Treated by CLDT physiotherapist while still in plaster
- Referred by orthopaedic consultant to a hand clinic—letter from hospital physiotherapist to CLDT physiotherapist left at home

- Telephone communication and liaison between physiotherapists
- *Secondary diagnosis*: Reflex sympathetic dystrophy (RSD)
- Hospital appointments not always kept; seriousness of condition explained to client, key worker, landlady and centre staff. Discussed with CLDT nurse
- Weekly exercises with physiotherapist at CLDT resource centre and return to country dancing. Hospital physiotherapy appointments kept with assistance from key worker and CLDT nurse.
- Three months later, discharged from hospital physiotherapist. Exercises continued at resource centre until full range of movements achieved.

The outcome

Went on to become a member of the country dance display team who danced at a conference and local country dance club.

The twenty-first century and future

The twenty-first century has already seen dramatic changes and developments in the thinking about the care and support of people with learning disabilities. Central to these changes are people with learning disabilities themselves. No longer are they prepared to passively accept care and services that do not meet their needs. People with learning disabilities are finding their voice and demanding a top seat at the decision-making table. They are demonstrating that their contribution is valid and their views are ones which must be heard to enable them to lead ordinary lives, with the necessary support required based upon individual need.

Policy makers have been busy. Devolution of government within Scotland brought the publication of 'The Same as You? A review of services for people with learning disabilities' (Scottish Executive, 2000). 'The Same as You?' is the blue print for services for children and adults with learning disabilities in

Scotland, and will shape care and support in the future. The report is built around seven key principles:

- People with learning disabilities should be valued. They should be asked and encouraged to contribute to the community in which they live
- People with learning disabilities are individual people
- People with learning disabilities should be asked about the services they need and be involved in making choices about what they want
- People with learning disabilities should be helped and supported to do everything they are able to do
- Wherever possible, people with learning disabilities should be helped to use the same local services as everyone else
- People with learning disabilities should benefit from specialist social, health and educational services
- People with learning disabilities should have services, which take account of their age, abilities and other needs.

A government implementation group is taking forward the recommendations within Scotland. The report contains significant recommendations that will see the closure of the remaining long-stay hospitals by 2005. The other recommendations brought about the establishment of the Scottish Consortium for Learning Disabilities that brings together 13 organisations concerned with the care and support of people with learning disabilities. Advocacy services, many already established, will also be developed to enable and support people with learning disabilities to have their voice heard and views taken into account. Another significant development is the establishment of Local Area Coordination, a concept that has been imported from Western Australia. Local Area Coordination seeks to support people within their local community and develop links locally. There is a significant recommendation that will take forward Direct Payments, which will enable people with learning disabilities to develop flexible supports to meet their needs, independently from those provided by statutory services. All long-stay hospital beds will go and, wherever possible, health care will be provided in a range of mainstream settings. The health service will develop models of care to support assessment and treatment of those with the most complex and challenging needs. Central to the development of services is joint commissioning, in a partnership between statutory services and voluntary organisations.

In July 2002, the Scottish Executive published 'Promoting Health, Supporting Inclusion: The national review of the contribution of all nurses and midwives to the care and support of people with learning disabilities'. The report is set within the context of the care and support of children and adults with learning disabilities within community settings, and the range of contributions that nurses and midwives from all nursing backgrounds need to make to improve the health and well-being of people with learning disabilities, as part of the drive towards addressing inequalities and supporting inclusion.

In 2001, the report 'Valuing People: A New Strategy for learning disability in the 21st Century' was published by the English Department of Health. The strategy is built on four key principles—Rights, Independence, Choice, and Inclusion. The strategy recognises that people with learning disabilities wish for control over their own lives and that carers often require additional support. Housing opportunities need to be developed further to ensure that there are appropriate choices available. Employment and paid work are seen as priority areas and it is estimated that less then ten percent of people with learning disabilities have jobs. The strategy recognises the need to improve the health of people with learning disabilities and states that services need to be built around the needs of the individual, and that additional specialist support needs to be available when required. A new role of **Health Facilitator** is recommended to help support people with learning disabilities receive the care they need. The strategy also recommends **Health Action Plans** should be available and form part of person-centred plans. The Health Action Plan should detail the interventions and support required. It is recommended that Health Facilitators should be in place for all people with learning disabilities by June 2003, and all should have a Health Action Plan by June 2005. 'Valuing People' contains 11 broad objectives, focussing on disabled children and young people, transition into adult life, more choice and control, supporting carers, good health, housing, fulfilling lives, moving into employment, quality, workforce planning, and partnership working.

Conclusion

This chapter has sought to highlight policy developments and changes that have impacted upon people with learning disabilities in the Western world. Many of the developments that have taken place were not based around the needs of people with learning disabilities. In some cases, they have been driven by fear and prejudice and, in others, by the desire to help and protect. Today there is an increasing recognition that people with learning disabilities are individuals, with the right to self-determination. Policy in the twenty-first century attempts to recognise this and ensure that opportunities are developed to support people with learning disabilities, so that they can be heard and influence decisions which impact upon their lives.

References

APA (1994) *DSM-IV Diagnostic and Statistical Manual of Mental Disorders*, 4th edn. American Psychiatric Association, Washington, DC

Allan P, Pahl J, Quine L (1990) *Care Staff in Transition—The Impact on Staff of Changing Services for People with Mental Handicaps*. HMSO, London

Bobath K, Bobath B (1975) *Motor Development in the Different Types of Cerebral Palsy*. Heineman, London

Brown J (1992) The residential setting in mental handicap: an overview of selected policy initiatives. In: Thompson T, Mathias P, eds. *Standards and Mental Handicap*. Bailliere Tindall, London: 106–22

Department of Health (2001) *Valuing People: A New Strategy for Learning Disability for the 21st Century*. The Stationery Office, Edinburgh

Department of Health (1998) Signposts for Success. In: *Commissioning and Providing Health Services for People with Learning Disabilities*. HMSO, London

Department of Health (1995) *The Health of the Nation—A Strategy for People with Learning Disabilities*. HMSO, London

Department of Health (1992) *The Health of the Nation*. HMSO, London

Department of Health (1989) *Caring for People: Community Care in the Next Decade and Beyond*. HMSO, London

Department of Health (1988) *Community Care: Agenda for Action* (Griffiths Report). HMSO, London

Department of Health and Social Security (1987) *Mental Handicap: Progress, Problems and Priorities: A Review of Mental Handicap Services in England since the 1971 White Paper 'Better Services for the Mentally Handicapped'*. HMSO, London

Department of Health and Social Security (1978) *Development Team for the Mentally Handicapped: First Report 1976–77*. HMSO, London

Department of Health and Social Security (1971) *Better Services for the Mentally Handicapped*. HMSO, London

Grossman HJ, ed (1973) *Manual on Terminology and Classification in Mental Retardation*. American Association on Mental Deficiency, Washington, DC

Hari M, Akos K (1988) *Conductive Education*. Routledge, London

Henderson Sir DK (1964) *The Evolution of Psychiatry in Scotland*. E and S Livingstone Ltd.

Kanner L (1964) *A History of the Care and Study of the Mentally Retarded*. Charles C Thomas Publisher, Springfield, Ill, USA

Kristiansen K, Ness NE (1987) *Hjelpesystenet: Igar, I dag I morgan*. The Occupational Therapy Department, Sör-Tröndelage University, Trondheim

Loudon JB (Chairman) (1992) *The Future of Mental Handicap Hospital Services in Scotland*. HMSO, Crown Copyright, Edinburgh

Mayston MJ (2002) Peopl*e with Cerebral Palsy: Effects of and Perspectives for* Therapy. *News Letter of British Association of Bobath Trained Therapists*: 40 1–23

Morris P (1969) *Put Away*. Routledge and Keegan Paul, London

Nirje B (1969) The Normalisation Principle and its human management implications. In: Kugel R, Wolfensberger W, eds. *Changing Patterns in Residential Services for the Mentally Retarded*.

President's Committee on Mental Retardation, Washington: 179–95(b)

Rennie J, ed (2001) *Learning Disability, Physical therapy, Treatment and Management*. Whurr Publishers, London

Scheerenberger RC (1987) *A History of Mental Retardation*. Paul H Brooks Publishing, Baltimore

Scottish Executive (2002) *Promoting Health, Supporting Inclusion: The National Review of the Contribution of all Nurses and Midwives to the Care and Support of People with Learning Disabilities*. The Stationery Office, Edinburgh

Scottish Executive (2000) *The Same as You? A Review of Services for People with Learning Disabilities*. The Stationery Office, Edinburgh

Scrivens E (1986) The National Health Service: origins and issues. In: Patrick DL, Scambler G, eds. *Sociology as Applied to Medicine*. Bailliere Tindall, London: 204–10

Tredgold AF (1909) The Feeble-Minded: A Social Danger. *Eugenics Rev* **1**(3): 155

Trent JW (1994) *Inventing the Feeble Mind—A History of Mental Retardation in the United States*. University of California Press, Berkeley, LA

Turner S, Sweeney D, Hayes L (1995) *Developments in Community Care for Adults with Learning Disabilities: A Review of 1993/94 Community Care Plans*. Hester Adrian Research Centre, University of Manchester, HMSO, London

Tyne A, O'Brien J (1981) *The Principles of Normalisation*. Campaign for Mentally Handicapped People/Campaign for Mental Handicap Education and Research Association. (CMH /CMHERA), London

United Nations Declaration on the Rights of Disabled Persons (1975) *General Assembly Resolution 3447* (XXX) of December 9,1975, UN, New York

United Nations Declaration on the Rights of Mentally Retarded Persons (1971) *General Assembly Resolution 2865* (XXVI) of December 20, 1971, UN, New York

Welsh Office (1983) *All Wales Strategy for the Development of Services for Mentally Handicapped People*. HMSO, London

WHO (1992) *The ICD 10 Classification of Mental and Behavioural Disorders. Clinical Descriptions and Diagnostic Guidelines*. World Health Organization, Geneva

WHO (1980) *The International Classification of Impairments, Disabilities and Handicaps*. World Health Organization, Geneva

Wolfensberger W (1992) *A Brief Introduction to Social Role Valorisation as a High-Order Concept for Structuring Human Services*, rev edn. Training Institute for Human Service Planning, Leadership and Changing Agentry (Syracuse University), Syracuse, NY

Wolfensberger W, Thomas S (1983) *PASSING (Programme Analysis of Service Systems' Implementation of Normalisation Goals): Normalisation Criteria and Ratings Manual*, 2nd edn. National Institute on Mental Retardation, Toronto

2
Addressing inequalities

Michael Brown and Douglas Paterson

What is health?

Health means different things to different people. Attempts to accurately offer a definition that is all encompassing can be problematic. To some, health may mean being fit enough to climb Mount Everest. To others, it might mean living with a condition, such as diabetes, and working to make sure that the potential complications are limited. Health might include the recognition of the impact that unemployment and poor housing can have on an individual, their family and the wider community in which they live. Health, therefore, can be considered from a wide number of perspectives: from the perspective of an individual, a family, a particular group, or population; through to whole countries and continents. What is also now recognised and accepted are, what is termed, health inequalities. Health inequalities exist across populations and include issues, such as, the impact of unemployment, pollution, increases in mortality (*the number of people who die over a period of time*), changes in morbidity (*the number of people with specific diseases or illnesses over a period of time*), gender, socio-economic status, lifestyle and behaviours. Whatever the health inequalities and the definitions adopted, all the issues that affect and influence health in the general population can and do impact on the lives of people with learning disabilities and their carers. In many cases, the impact and consequences of health inequalities have a profound effect and may be life long.

Nearly half a century ago, the World Health Organization conceptualised health, broadly taking account of the multiple domains of human life and its enrichment. This approach may be somewhat surprising considering the Western medical model's preoccupation with disease treatment, or even prevention. By developing and broadening the definition, the complexity of health as not just an issue that requires to be addressed by doctors and health services emerged. Health is seen as a complex matrix of issues, circumstances and situations, the origins of which are often outwith the direct personal control of the individual. A strong and prosperous economy, for example, leads to improved employment opportunities which, in turn, has an important influence on health and well being. Having or not having a job can, therefore, be seen as having a significant impact upon health.

The World Health Organization's (1958) much quoted definition of health continues to be valid today:

> *'A state of complete physical, mental and social well-being and not merely the absence of disease or infirmity'.*

The humanist, Maslow (1971), put forward a hierarchical structure about how these health components are organised, with lower order elements needing to be fulfilled before achieving those that are higher. The term 'self-actualisation' was used to describe how it is necessary to fulfil the lower order needs, to work through the hierarchy of needs to achieve a state of fulfilment, **self-actualisation**. As a member of society, everyone has these potential needs and the opportunity to experience their achievement—including people with learning disabilities. When thinking about Maslow's model in relation to the general population, few people reach the apex—complete self actualisation. The majority, however, can fulfil their lower levels of needs. For some people with learning disabilities, achieving this level can prove difficult, and considerable additional support and care is necessary. This point is important when thinking about people with learning disabilities, as the level of intellectual impairment and associated disability increases with the severity of the learning disability. Maslow's model remains a helpful tool today when considering needs and aspirations.

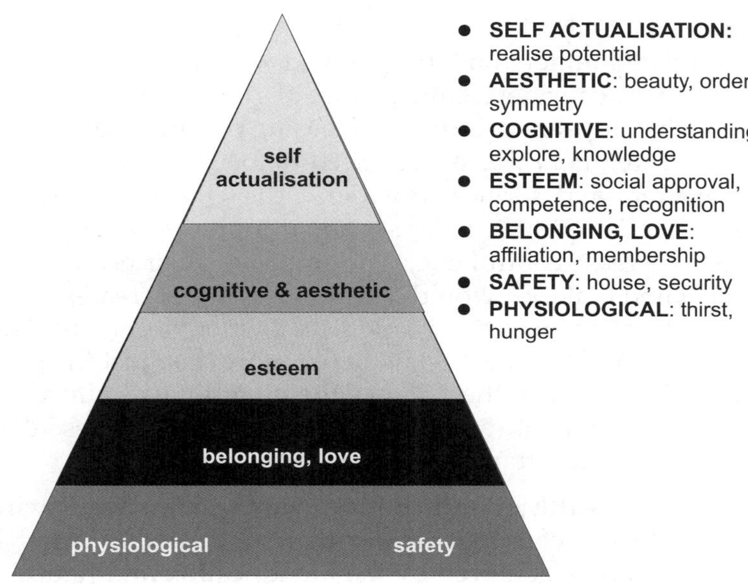

Figure 2.1: Abraham Maslow—Hierarchy of needs

Contemporary researchers, such as Jenkins (1992), have moved the work forward by reconceptualising these ideas to include issues, such as, **quality of life** and **subjective health**, in a move towards defining and understanding the more complex notion of health. This has followed decades where health has been judged in terms of behaviour change, cognitive change or physical and mental pathology.

A shift in focus—the recognition of inequalities

In 1980, the Black Report was first published, and was a landmark in the understanding of the complex and multiple issues that affected and impacted upon health within the United Kingdom. The report pointed to and identified the marked inequalities in health across and between the different social classes. Although it is approaching twenty-five years since the report was first published, it is important to note that, while the determinants of health and the inequalities are more fully recognised and understood, the gap had widened, not closed.

When first considering the picture of gross health inequalities and what appears to be ever increasing consumer demands for health care, there was a clear need to focus the activities of policy makers and service providers. The *Ottawa Charter for Health Promotion* (WHO, 1986) set about a process of enabling people to increase control over, and improve, their health. The Charter stated that they would need to identify and realise their aspirations, satisfy needs and cope with their environment. The improvement of health was considered more than just the goal of the health sector; rather, it was the co-ordinated efforts of different government and private agencies. The essential components of the Ottawa Charter included:

1. **Building Healthy Public Policy:** making all sectors aware of the health consequences of their policies and actions. This would be achieved by the identification and removal of obstacles by taxation, legislation and organisational change;
2. **Creating Supportive Environments:** with the guiding principle of reciprocal maintenance to help change patterns of life, work and leisure so that they are safe, stimulating, satisfying and enjoyable;
3. **Strengthen Community Actions:** empowering communities to take ownership and control of their destinies, which are locally determined, planned and acted upon;
4. **Develop Personal Skills:** through information, education for health and enhancing life skills. By doing so, to enable people to learn throughout life to prepare for all stages and challenges of life in a more constructive way; and
5. **Reorient Health Services:** to more than just the provision of clinical and curative services. This would include a change of attitude and organisation of health services within the broader changes of the social, political and economical environment.

Nearly two decades later, in 1998, the *Independent Inquiry into Inequalities in Health Report* was completed by Sir Donald Acheson in the United Kingdom. The report stated that it remains clear that, as we move into the twenty-first century, inequalities in health continue to exist irrespective of the measures used. The inequalities experienced impact on and affect the whole of society across the life span. It also highlighted the key issues that impact on and contribute to inequalities, and includes poverty, income, tax and benefits, education, employment, housing and environment, mobility, transport and pollution, and nutrition. The areas identified support the view that, while health care services and workers have an important role to play in promoting health and providing health care, there are significant other areas that are key contributors to the inequalities experienced. To address such wide and far-reaching issues, political action and determination is necessary, both in health care and in other policy areas in order to even begin to make an impact. Three main areas are identified as crucial in order to take this forward:

- All policies areas, such as **housing and state benefits** that impact on health, need to be evaluated to determine the extent to which they do, in fact, impact on and reduce health inequalities over time
- A high priority needs to be given to improving the health and wealth of **children and families**
- Action needs to be taken, via the state **taxation system,** that seeks to reduce income inequalities and improve the living standards of the poorest and most disadvantaged.

In 2002, the report *Securing Our Future Health: Taking a Long-Term View*, (often referred to as *The Wanless Report* after the chair of the report's working group, Derek Wanless) was published by the British Treasury. This report was a far reaching review of the spending required on health care over the next 20 years and identified the need for increased health spending as a result of increasing needs, the need to address changing demographics, the need to improve information technology within health care, and enhance the skills of health care professionals and the role of primary care services.

The World Health Organization (2002) published *The European Health Report,* as part of the requirement to publish public health information relevant to the member states within Europe. The WHO European Health Report seeks to build a healthy population and tackle ill health. This will be achieved, in part, by reducing mortality, morbidity and disability within the poorest and most marginalised populations. Central to this aim is the need to promote healthy lifestyles and limit the risks to health that can be associated with environmental, economic, social and behavioural causes. The role of health services is identified in relation to the need to develop equitable health care systems that improve the outcomes for those with the greatest need. It is now recognised that people with learning disabilities access primary care services with a similar frequency to the general population. Considering their greater needs, a greater frequency could be anticipated (Whitfield *et al,* 1996). The pivotal role of primary health is given prominence and supports the view that strategies aimed at addressing inequalities and improving health should be driven from there. All these issues impact upon people with learning disabilities who, despite living longer and the improvements in mortality, still continue to die sooner when compared with the general population (Hollins *et al,* 1998). It is now well established that, while the life expectancy of people with learning disabilities has increased overall, it remains shorter in absolute terms (Strauss and Eyman, 1996).

Equity

A vision that seeks to promote equity for all must be set within the context of the wider determinants of health and well being, and must take account of core issues, such as poverty, employment, education, lifestyles, the physical environment, and the provision of effective health systems and health care. The World Health Organization has considered the concept of **health equity** and states that, when looking at health, wider moral and ethical issues arise that must also be taken in to account. **Health inequity** refers to and takes account of differences between groups that are unnecessary and, as a result, could be avoidable and preventable. These situations can be described as **unfair and unjust** and, therefore, require to be addressed. They go on to state:

> *'In order to describe a certain situation as inequitable, the cause has to be examined and judged to be unfair in the context of what is going on in the rest of society'*
>
> (Whitehead, 1990)

Within the endeavour to bridge, what is now being recognised as, health divides among populations, multiple tactics need to be employed. Considering the wide range of health needs, the overall policy aim is to seek to improve the health of the country by promoting equity for all people. This, in turn, impacts upon the general health of the whole population. The idea of promoting and improving public health is not new, and social and public health reformers in the nineteenth century, for example, brought about changes and improvements in general hygiene,

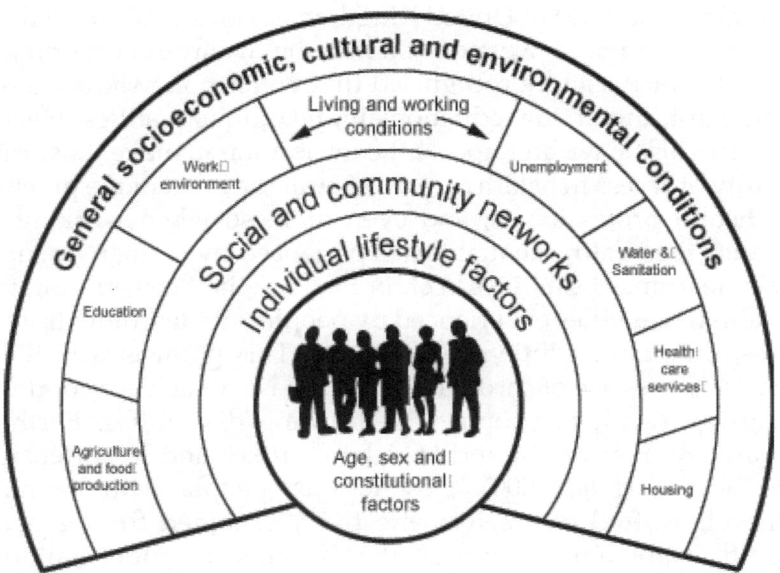

Figure 2.2: The Determinants of Health from Dahlgren and Whithead, 1991

nutrition, and accommodation that, when considered retrospectively, demonstrates an increase in the average life expectancy of the general population. Such changes and improvements in health inequalities can be seen in line with the fall of major diseases, such as tuberculosis, and predating the effects of modern medical treatments, such as antibiotics. This means that wider efforts to identify, address, and reduce health inequalities and improve health will require a longer-term investment that must be tracked over time in order to see the benefits.

In identifying the wider determinants of health inequalities, it is important to recognise the specific role of health care systems and services in the drive to improve health and reduce health inequalities. Across the Western world, health services are funded by a range of methods, often a mix of taxation and private health insurance. Within the United Kingdom, the founding principle of the National Health Service in 1948 was one of a service free at the point of delivery, and one that promoted equity in access to all citizens. These principles remain at the heart of United Kingdom governments, in all their devolved forms, as we move on into the twenty-first century.

It is increasingly recognised that wider policy impacts on, and can bring about reductions in, health inequalities. Health services also have an important contribution to make. Ensuring equity of access to health care must be at the heart of the practice of health professionals, and even more so when working to reduce the health inequalities experienced by so many people with learning disabilities. Yet, in reality, when considering the health inequalities experienced by people with learning disabilities, they attract little specific focus. This point is well illustrated in the case of coronary heart disease, which is a common cause of death in people with learning disabilities. Further, many are overweight and at risk of strokes and hypertension (Robertson *et al*, 2000). Despite this, people with learning disabilities find themselves effectively excluded from general health campaigns, without the benefits of more tailored approaches.

In recognition of the wider determinants of health, there is increasing emphasis on the need to ensure that effective local planning and collaboration among health, social services, and the voluntary sector is in place. Within the area of learning disabilities, strategies to improve the lives of people with learning disabilities place increasing importance on joint working between agencies, as well as with service users, families and carers.

People with learning disabilities: addressing inequalities

People with learning disabilities form a heterogeneous group and often find themselves members of the most disadvantaged in society. They are distributed throughout all groups and social classes and, as with all groups within society, have everyday needs. Everyday needs, such as, the need to be safe, warm, have food, and shelter—the very things identified by Maslow that, today, seem basic and often taken for granted. Following on from this is the need for people with learning disabilities to form and develop loving relationships and be recognised as individuals, who all have distinct qualities and contributions to make. Today, people with learning disabilities are increasingly becoming their own best advocates, as they begin to state clearly and effectively their right to be visible and be heard. Their desire to lead full and inclusive lives is reflected in their demand for ordinary lives. As with others, all people with learning disabilities have health needs. There is an increasing body of knowledge that highlights how, for a significant number, their basic health needs—those taken for granted by many—are not being identified and met. These needs are discussed more fully in a later chapter.

The health needs of people with learning disabilities can be considered from three perspectives:

- Everyday health needs applicable to anyone in the general population

- Additional health needs resulting from having a learning disability
- Additional health needs resulting from the specific cause of the learning disability, often described as complex needs. People with this level of need also have everyday health needs.

All people with learning disabilities have everyday health needs, which includes: the need for immunisation as a child, and hearing and vision tests. In order for everyday health needs to be assessed and met, it is necessary to have access to health care workers—doctors, nurses, therapist, pharmacists, etc, who are familiar with everyday health issue, as well as those found in people with learning disabilities. For others, there will be health needs that result because of the learning disability. More specific health needs that are found in some people with learning disabilities are considered in other chapters of this book, including the increase in psychiatric illness and genetic issues.

Research in the area of learning disabilities overall remains low when considered in relation to that undertaken in areas, such as, coronary heart disease and cancers. There is a need to ensure that people with learning disabilities are considered and included in 'mainstream' health research studies, as well as in studies that look for specific ways to improve their health. The limited focus exposes a significant gap in the knowledge and understanding of the additional help and support that is required by people with learning disabilities (Horwitz *et al*, 2000). The need to study the health inequalities experienced by people with learning disabilities and the impact on mortality and morbidity is essential, if the efforts aimed at improving their health are to be effective.

In reality, the health inequalities that have been experienced by people with learning disabilities have, according to Espie and Brown (1998), been the subject of what is describe as 'myths'. The myths centre around the misconception that people with learning disability have good health and that health services can and do address their needs effectively. This has, in part, come about through a desire to avoid labelling and the accusation of over medicalisation, but has, in effect, resulted in denial of the true extent of the health needs of people with learning disabilities. To tackle these issues, the focus of health services must be to fully address health gaps and inequalities that exist *'in as exemplary a way as other inequalities'* (Espie and Brown, 1998: 606). Such recognition is not restricted to the United Kingdom.

In New Zealand, there has been a focus on health screening that, as with other countries, identified significant health inequalities (Beange *et al*, 1995; Webb and Rogers, 1999). The publication of 'Closing the Gap' in 2002 by the Surgeon General in the United States highlighted that, while the needs of every person with a learning disability are unique, the need for effective, active health care is real and, in practice, goes unrecognised and, therefore, unmet. The blueprint sets out goals that state:

- **Goal 1**: Integrate health promotion into the community environments of people with learning disabilities
- **Goal 2**: Increase knowledge and understanding of health and learning disabilities, ensuring that knowledge is made practical and easy to use
- **Goal 3**: Improve the quality of health care for people with learning disabilities
- **Goal 4**: Train health care providers in the care of adults and children with learning disabilities
- **Goal 5**: Ensure that health care financing produces good health outcomes for adults and children with learning disabilities
- **Goal 6**: Increase sources of health care for adults, adolescents and children with learning disabilities, ensuring that health care is easily accessible.

The increasing recognition is important when considering the increasing longevity of the lives of people with learning disabilities, as an increase in life expectancy will bring with it increasing numbers of diseases experienced, such as cancers (Hogg *et al*, 2001), and other ill health associated with living longer. When considering improvements in the life expectancy for people with learning disabilities, those with Downs's syndrome are a good example. Their life expectancy has dramatically increased over the twentieth century, albeit still being less than the general population. This point is well demonstrated by Yang *et al* (2002), who used data from US death certificates over a 14-year period. Of nearly 18 000 people studied with Down's syndrome, they noted a jump in median age at death from 25 in 1983 to 49 in 1997. This said, there remains a significant gap in life expectancy when people with learning disabilities are compared with the general population, with the average at birth being from 74 to 76.5 years. It is now recognised that life expectancy of people with learning disability decreases as the severity of the learning disability and physical disability increases (Janicki *et al*, 1999). Recognising such changes over time

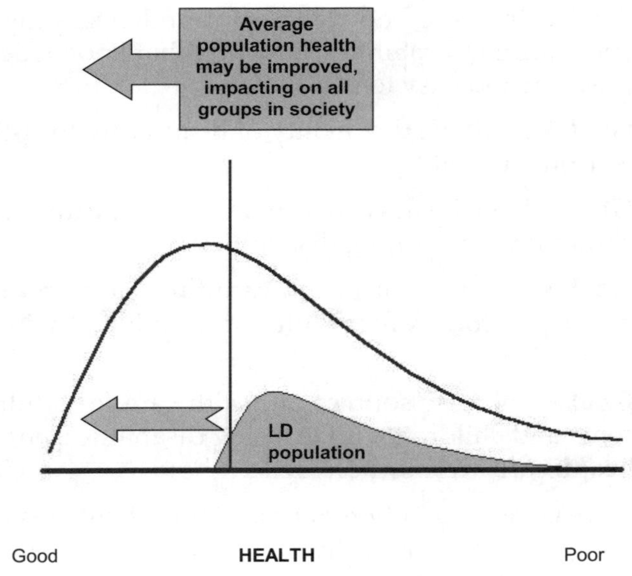

Figure 2.3: Tactics to improve health

is important, as it is likely that overall longevity will increase for people with learning disabilities, which will lead to an increasing number living on into old age. As a result, there is a need to focus on the needs of those who live longer and often present with co-morbidity of multiple health needs that are 'layered' on each other.

Reducing inequalities and promoting health

Over the past two decades, improving health has formed a key component of government strategies for both the general population and people with learning disabilities. Before this, there had been little specific attention given to improving health. The Department of Health published the *Health of the Nation* in 1992 that identified the need to focus on health inequality priority areas, such as, mental health, coronary heart disease, cancers, strokes, AIDS and HIV, and accidents. *The Health of the Nation: A Strategy for People with Learning Disabilities* was developed in 1995 and adopted the priority areas outlined in the *Health of the Nation*. In 1998, the focus on the need to consider the poor health experienced by some people with learning disabilities also led to the publication, by the Department of Health, of *Signposts for Success*. This sought to inform and guide the commissioning of health services for people with learning disabilities. The International Association of the Scientific Study of Intellectual Disabilities (IASSID) has developed guidelines and recommendations aimed at reducing health inequalities (Beange *et al*, 1999). Their recommendations have been referred to the World Health Organization for adoption.

Strategies seeking to improve health need to be built on the foundations of evidence-based practise. MacIntyre (2003) notes the lack of good research in areas of public policy. In particular, the area of intervention effectiveness, where Milward *et al* (2001) find only four percent of public health research concerning itself with interventions and 0.4% with the outcome of interventions. While pharmacological research has flourished in this medium, large-scale research looking at strategies to affect health inequalities has not been undertaken to the same extent.

To date within the arena of research into the needs of people with learning disabilities, the evidence that exists is, according Horwitz *et al* (2000), lacking in the consistent methodologies needed to enable effective comparison.

In part, this situation rests with the difficulties of studying complex ecosystems. Whether describing the health needs, risks

An individual focus on:

1. Lifestyle risk analysis:
   - *Smoking*
   - *Drinking*
   - *Diet*
   - *Exercise*
   - *Sexual behaviour*
2. Genetic profiles
3. Medical examination and investigations
4. Cognitive mediators:
   - *Locus of control, Rotter (1966)*
   - *Attitudes*
   - *Risk perception.*

Whole populations focussing on:

1. Barriers to unhealthy behaviour:
   - *Tobacco and alcohol higher taxation*
   - *License restriction of alcohol*
   - *Restriction of smoking places*
   - *Regulating advertising of tobacco.*
2. Promoting healthy behaviour:
   - *Farming/food subsidies*
   - *Targeted discounts, e.g. sport membership*
   - *Targeted subsidy, e.g. Winter fuel allowance*
   - *Free barrier contraception*
   - *Labelling products, eg smoking, food.*
3. Promoting attitude change:
   - *School education programs*
   - *Media advertising campaigns*
   - *Influencing TV/cinema stereotypes.*

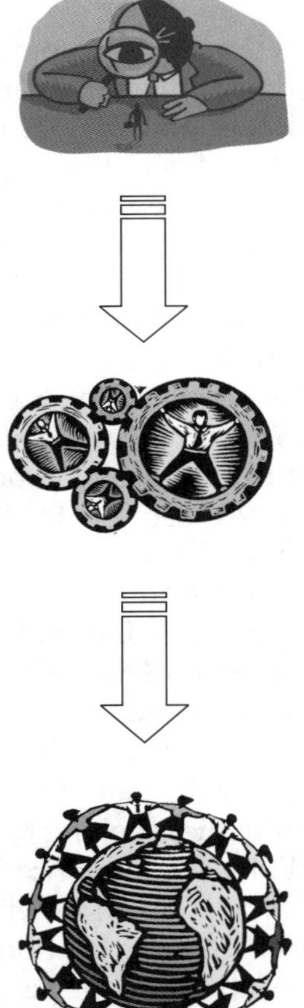

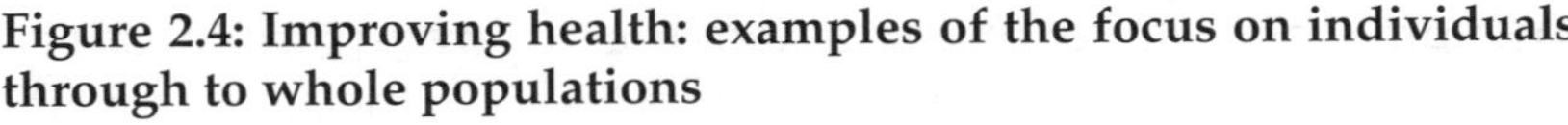

Figure 2.4: Improving health: examples of the focus on individuals through to whole populations

and inequalities, or examining the impact of a therapeutic intervention, the focus can be from the micro to the macro-environment, and everything in between. A therapist might concentrate on a single person with learning disabilities, characterising health behaviours, current disease state, risk or morbidity, then design and test interventions and treatments before assessing how effective these were. By contrast, government allocation of funding would consider the wider perspective of large groups or whole population, with their need for treatment, additional benefits or standing in the community. Campaigns might be nationally based in the media or through changing laws.

Considering models to improve health

Different funding and organisational structures exist within services—health, education, and social services across the world, and within countries. This is understandable when considered in the context of local need and geography—large inner cities through to island rural and remote areas, with structures reflecting the needs of the population served. When health services are examined, they present a complex picture of community-based services through to university teaching hospitals that provide highly specialised services, often on a region-wide basis. An evolving model to consider the complexities is developing in the shape of a 'Tiered Model of Care'. The Tiered Model is attracting attention, as it is one way to conceptualise complex systems and organisations and see the inter-relatedness across all the Tiers and the importance of their contributions to care (Scottish Executive, 2002). At Tier 0, the first tier, services are more widely available to all at a community level, meeting the mass of needs. Higher Tiers, 1 and 2, have gatekeepers, such as GPs, to restrict access by way of referral to the Tiers above. Some services, such as regional neurology and cancer care centres, through to secure forensic units, are required by relatively few individuals, and are usually expensive in terms of beds and workers who possess specialist knowledge. Such health services are often shared across larger areas and aim to treat those with the most complex and challenging needs.

Goldberg and Huxley (1980) studied the access for people with mental illness to different services. They described the existence of **filters**, which influenced access to services. A key issue arising from their work was the fact that the filters operated not just to direct *appropriate* healthcare, but also in a

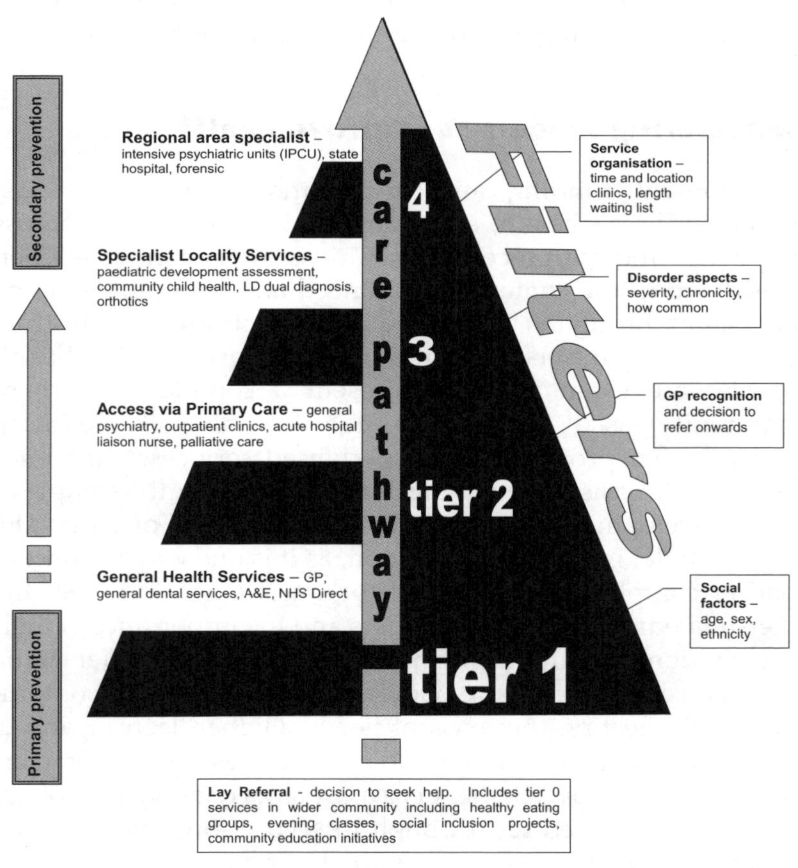

Figure 2.5: The Tier Model of Care

negative way. It is now recognised that people with learning disabilities experience barriers when accessing health (Lennox *et al*, 1997). The barriers take the form of physical ones, such as limited access to a health centre, as the result of being wheelchair bound, communication barriers, and the inability to access health care due to the perception that a person with a learning disability is incapable of giving informed consent to a medical procedure. Often, at the core of many barriers are important fundamental issues, such as insufficient training and experience of the needs of people with learning disabilities, which limits recognition of their problems, to more insidious problems arising from prejudice and stereotyping. The issue of subtle discrimination and prejudice exists for people with learning disabilities in areas of healthcare, where topics may be sensitive and awkward, as in sexual health. People with learning disabilities are sexually active and, therefore, require access to appropriate sexual health care. In other situations, it is now recognised that some people with learning disabilities will be the victims of sexual abuse (Sosbey *et al*, 1991), and access to sexual health care and counselling is necessary. It is now acknowledged that women with learning disabilities are more likely to be excluded from national cervical screening campaigns (Pearson *et al*, 1998).

When considering the issue of prevention and the limitation of ill health, and the interface of services between and across the different tiers, the greatest potential impact on the learning disability population lies in the primary prevention of illness at the lower tiers. By the time people reach the higher tiers, where secondary prevention may operate, morbidity has already started to take effect. The major focus, therefore, needs to be on prevention and support at a primary care level.

Trying to collate the multiple factors that impact on and affect health needs within the context of service systems is complex. Conceptualised models are a way of trying to address these issues and the work of Tansella and Thornicroft (1999) suggest a **Matrix Model**. The Matrix Model is a helpful way of enabling direct health and social care workers, planners and commissioners of services to make 'sense' of a wide range of complex elements that are interrelated. The Matrix Model offers two dimensions—***geographical***, which is further divided in to three levels: country [1], local [2] and patient [3], and the ***temporal*** dimension—inputs [A], process [B] and outcomes [C]. Within the Matrix Model the authors denote grouped elements as ***cells***. Some cells in the model will include issues that might not be routinely considered and recognised as having an influence and, hence, need to be taken into account. An example of this would be the cell that contains media influences. Such images and influences are outwith the control of service providers, yet can have a significant impact. The significance of the press and media and their impact—positive and negative—are often over looked when considering the factors that impact on health. An example from the book, *Media Madness: Public Images of Mental Illness,* by Wahl (1995) illustrates the point and notes that:

> *'People with mental illnesses are also readers and viewers of those images; they are shamed by them and they're embarrassed by them. They're aware that they are depicted in negative ways and it damages their self-esteem, it damages their confidence, and it increases the likelihood that they won't tell anyone about their illnesses. So they're not going to seek treatment.'*

In practise, the 'Matrix Model' provides a way of understanding how the multiple inequalities might, for example, affect a health care worker undertaking an individual needs assessment (*cell 3A*). The cell might refer to a hospital or social work service, operational policies, and pathways to care; (*cell 2B*) for guidance on their actions. The issue of case management could be considered in *cell 2B* and may determine the length of time a worker might spend with a service user, thereby influencing the quality of treatment (*cell 3B*). The interventions have the potential to influence and bring about a greater or lesser symptom reduction (*cell 3C*), which in turn affects the burden on caregivers. An alternative application of the Matrix Model is a scenario where a worker provides a service to users in central London compared to the rural Highlands of Scotland (*cell 2A*), with different population characteristics and services available.

		TEMPORAL DIMENSION		
		A–Input Phase	B–Process Phase	C–Outcome Phase
GEOGRAPHICAL DIMENSION	1. Country/ Region Level	**Cell 1A** • Expenditure on services • Role of media • Mental health law • Government directives • Special interest groups	**Cell 1B** • Performance activity indicators, e.g. admission rates, bed occupancy rates, compulsory treatment rates	**Cell 1C** • Suicide rates • Standardised Mortality Rate • Homelessness • Special enquiries
	2. Local Level	**Cell 2A** • Population needs assessment • Population characteristics • Budget • Staff • Fixed expenditure • Consumer participation	**Cell 2B** • Operational policies • Pathways to care • Patterns of service use • Case loads • Targeting of special groups	**Cell 2C** • Outcome studies at group level • Secondary and tertiary prevention • Decrease of local stigma • Better access to services
	3. Individual Level	**Cell 3A** • Individual needs assessment • Demands made by patient • Demands made by families	**Cell 3B** • quality of treatments • Frequency and duration of treatment • Continuity of care • Income support • Vocational services	**Cell 3C** • Symptom reduction • Satisfaction • Quality of life/ accommodatio n • Disability/work rehabilitation • Burdon on caregivers

Figure 2.6: The Matrix Model, adapted from Thornicroft and Tansella (1999)

From a country point of view, differences may exist as they respond to alternative outcomes *(cell 1C and 3C)*, perhaps in response to a specific enquiry; and in an attempt to action change by financial incentives, government directives or laws, (*cell 1A*). Another examples is in social and attitudinal changes over time, (*cell 1A*), which has the potential to modulate all other factors, often stimulated by special interest groups or experienced through the media.

Historically, people with learning disabilities have been a neglected group within society and have poorer health than other groups. People with learning disabilities are demanding to be seen as people first and wish to be recognised as individuals, with unique and distinct needs. There is an increasing body of evidence suggesting that the ordinary health needs of people with learning disabilities are a neglected area and, as a result, many experience unmet health needs and live with the consequences.

There is increasing recognition of the need to address inequalities in health across countries and increasing focus on the wider determinants of health and ill health along the factors that impact on and affect them. Policy today is seeking to identify and redress these inequalities, an effort that requires intervention beyond that of health care services alone. In the past, people with learning disabilities have been given a limited focus in health research and there is a need to ensure they are included in work that is undertaken in the future. Actively considering and including people with learning disabilities, and ensuring they are visible within strategies aimed at improving health, will begin to have an impact on what has been one of our most disadvantaged groups.

References

Beange H, Lennox NG, Parmenter T (1999) Health targets for people with intellectual disability. *J Intell Dev Disabil* **24**(4): 283–97

Beange H, McElduff A, Baker W (1995) Medical disorders in adults with intellectual disability: a population study. *Am J Ment Retard* **99**(7): 595–604

Dahlgren G, Whitehead M (1991) *Policies and strategies to promote social equity in health.* World Health Organization, Geneva

Department of Health (1998) *Signposts for Success in Commissioning and Providing Services for People with Learning Disabilities*. HMSO, London

Department of Health (1995) *The Health of the Nation: A Strategy for People with Learning Disabilities.* HMSO, London

Department of Health (1992) *The Health of the Nation.* HMSO, London

Department of Health and Social Security (1980) *Inequalities in Health: The Black Report* HMSO, London

Espie C, Brown M (1998) Health needs and learning disabilities: An Overview. *Health Bull* **56**(2): 603–11

Goldberg D, Huxley P (1980) *Mental Illness in the Community: The Pathways to Psychiatric Care*. Tavistock Publications, London

Hogg J, Northfield J, Turnbull J, (2001) *Cancer and People with Learning Disabilities—The Evidence from Published Studies and Experiences from Cancer Services.* British Institute of Learning Disabilities, London

Hollins S, Attard MT, von Fraunhofer N, Sedgwick P (1998) Mortality in people with learning disabilities: risk, causes and death certification findings in London. *Dev Med Child Neurol* **40**: 50–56

Horwitz S, Kerker B, Owens P, Zigler P (2000) *The Health Status and Needs of Individuals with Mental Retardation.* Yale University Press, London and New York

HM Treasury (2002) *Securing Our Future Health: Taking a Long-Term View.* HMSO, London

Independent Inquiry into Inequalities in Health (1998) HMSO, London

Janicki MP, Dalton AJ, Henderson CM, Davidson PW (1999) Mortality and morbidity among older adults with intellectual disabilities: Health service considerations. *Disabil Rehab* **21**: 284–94

Jenkins CD (1992) Assessment of outcomes of health intervention. *Soc Sci Med* **35**: 367–75

Lennox N, Diggens J, Ugoni AM (1997) The general practice of the care of people with intellectual disability: barriers and solutions. *J Intellect Disabil Res* **41**: 380–90

MacIntyre S (2003) Evidence based policymaking: impact on health inequalities still needs to be assessed. *Br Med J* **326**: 5–6

Maslow A (1971) *The Farther Reaches of Human Nature*. The Viking Press, New York

Milward L, Kelly M, Nutbeam D (2001) *Public Health Intervention Research: The Evidence*. Health Development Agency, London

Pearson V, Davis C, Rouff C, Dyer J (1998) Only one quarter of women with learning disabilities in Exeter have cervical screening. *Br Med J* **316**: 1979

Robertson J, Emerson E, Gregory N, Hatton C, Kessisoglou S, Hallam A (2000) Lifestyle related risk factors for poor health in residential settings for people with intellectual disabilities. *Res Devel Disabil* **21**: 469–86

Rotter JB (1966) Generalised expectancies for internal and external control of reinforcement. *Psycholog Mon* **80**(609): 1–28

Scottish Executive (2002) *Promoting Health, Supporting Inclusion: The National Review of the Contribution of all Nurses and Midwives to the Care and Support of People with Learning Disabilities*. The Stationery Office, Edinburgh

Sosbey D, Gray S, Wells D (1991) *Disability and Abuse: An Annotated Bibliography*. Paul H Brooks, Baltimore

Strauss D, Eyman R (1996) Mortality of people with mental retardation in California with and without Down Syndrome, 1986–1991. *Am J Ment Retard* **100**(6): 643–53

Thornicroft G, Tansella M (1999) *The Mental Health Matrix: A Manual to Improve Services*. Cambridge University Press, Cambridge

United States Department of Health and Human Services (2002) *Closing the Gap: A National Blueprint to improve the healthcare of persons with mental retardation.* US Public Health Services, Washington, DC

Wahl OF (1995) *Media Madness: Public Images of Mental Illness.* Rutgers University Press, New Brunswick, NJ

Webb O, Rogers L (1999) Health screening for people with intellectual disability: the New Zealand experience. *J Intellect Disabil Res* **43**(6): 497–503

Whitfield M, Langan J, Russell O (1996) Assessing general practitioners' care of adults patients with learning disabilities: case control study. *Q Health Care* **5**: 31–35

World Health Organization (2002) *The European Health Report.* WHO Regional Publications: European series No. 97. WHO, Geneva

World Health Organization (1986) *Ottawa Charter for Health Promotion*. WHO, Geneva

World Health Organization (1958) *The First Ten Years. The Health Organisation*. WHO, Geneva

Yang Q, Rasmussen SA, Friedman JM (2002) Mortality associated with Down's syndrome in the USA from 1983 to 1997: a population-based study. *Lancet* **359**: 1019–25

3 Listening and including people with learning disabilities

Lisa Curtice

This chapter considers how services are changing to give people with learning disabilities and their families a greater say in developments that affect their lives. Two theoretical perspectives inform the discussions in this chapter. First, developments are located within current debates about the social model of disability and its relevance to people with learning disabilities. Second, the relationship between integration and inclusion is explored. A variety of opportunities to promote control and participation are identified. Developments in policy and practice within Scotland provide case study material. Finally, throughout the chapter, policy and practice are tested for robustness with respect to how far they touch the lives of people with profound and multiple disabilities.

Theoretical and historical perspectives

The chapter begins by considering some of the key philosophical debates underpinning recent service developments and the role of users' voices within these.

The social model of disability

The social model of disability refers to a political and social analysis of the causes and nature of disability, which states that disability is a consequence of the barriers erected by society, to the full participation of disabled people and, not necessarily, a self-limiting characteristic of having an impairment, such as not being able to see, hear, or walk on legs (Swain *et al*, 1993). In other words, the problem is everyone's responsibility and not the fault of the individual who has an impairment. The social model of disability is contrasted with 'the medical model', which refers to an individualistic analysis of disability, and seeks to tackle the issue by attempting, exclusively, to modify the person's impairment.

The social model arose out of the experiences of disabled people, of being segregated in residential establishments, denied the freedom to control their own lives and subject to humiliating interventions in the name of therapy (Campbell and Oliver, 1996). The social model is now widely accepted as a non-negotiable position across disability groups. Along the way, it has been necessary to recognise that impairments, while not explaining disability, do have specific consequences for people's lives; that oppression can undermine psycho-emotional well-being and that there are differences, as well as similarities, of experiences within the constituency of disabled people, including people of different genders, ethnic groups and relative social power (Thomas, 1999).

The issue of language has been of huge importance within disability politics, because language can be used to take away people's identity and legitimacy and to reinforce their exclusion from society and from power. Thus, within the disability movement, the word 'disability' is restricted to the limiting consequences of societal barriers, whereas a characteristic, such as, not being able to see, or to walk, is described as an 'impairment'. This distinction is seen as very important because it stresses that impairment should not lead to disability and exclusion. However, people with disabilities have claimed the term 'disabled people' as a mark of pride and solidarity. The disability movement has also emphasised an individual's right to the services he/she needs to lead an independent life in society. Thus, in describing services, the term 'support' or 'supports' is preferred to 'care'.

As Mark Priestley (1998) has shown, there are different strands within the social model perspective. The materialist approach emphasises the importance of power inequalities in structuring the lives of disabled people, whereas the idealist approach emphasises the ways in which images and language construct the disabled person as a threat and someone outside society (or even humanity). In material terms, people with learning disabilities experience huge inequalities because of the barriers that exclude them not only from employment, but also from the structure of the benefits and welfare system. From a cultural standpoint, the analysis is equally robust. People with learning disabilities have been 'labelled'; that is, excluded from opportunities for education, employment, social participation, and all the attributes of adult status because of assumptions about limited capacity and discriminatory stereotypes associated with their disability. Their emotional and spiritual needs have often been neglected (Curtice, 2001). People with learning disabilities are individuals with as diverse a range of capacities and needs as any other social group. Goodley (2001) has pointed out that, when people with learning disabilities can tell their own stories, they can oppose the 'tragic label' with images of resilience. Terms such as 'mental retardation' have been rejected as stigmatising because of the implication that the person will be unable to learn or grow up. In the UK, self advocates have preferred the term 'learning difficulties' because it emphasises that people have a continuing capacity to learn.

In particular, people with learning disabilities have been marginalised and excluded because of their lack of 'voice'; i.e., of the opportunity to express their views powerfully, to have their views treated with respect, and to see those views being taken account of, even in services that are set up with the intention of meeting their needs. An example of discrimination in this respect would be failing to ask a person with learning disabilities their views because they were perceived to have 'communication difficulties'. An approach grounded in the social model of disability would consider that person's access to communication support, whether in the form of access to speech therapy, a supporter or advocate, or alternative and augmentative communication aids.

There is a tension, even in distinguishing people with learning disabilities within the constituency of disabled people, because this may be seen to reinforce their identification through their impairment, to replicate their social and service experience by separating them off as different. On the other hand, it can be argued that to deny people with learning disabilities, the same opportunities to identify and reflect upon their circumstances as other disabled people, is to continue to deny them an important tool for their own empowerment.

Integration and inclusion

In order to respond to the changes required to end institutional living and practices, Wolfensberger developed the highly influential theory of normalisation, later revised as social role valorisation (1983). Normalisation principles sought to counter the effects of segregation by equalising the life circumstances and chances of people with learning disabilities with the rest of society. Popularised in the UK by the King's Fund as 'ordinary life' principles, normalisation theory emphasised the importance of people with learning disabilities being able to live in ordinary houses, with access to the same community facilities and social opportunities as everyone else (King's Fund Centre, 1980). In developing 'social role valorisation' theory, Wolfensberger acknowledged that it was not sufficient for the progress of such a marginalised group for them to be have equivalent opportunities. He argued that to reverse their stigmatisation and marginalisation, they would need to adopt particularly valued roles within society so that attitudes and norms would change.

Normalisation has been criticised as leading to integration rather than inclusion, adapting the disabled person to the societal norm rather than changing that norm to create a society in which disabled people play their full part. For example, integration might involve making special arrangements for someone to attend a club and then take part as much as they can in the activities of other members. An approach based in social inclusion would consider how the activity of the club could be shaped to be accessible to all those who might want to take part. Integration assumes that giving everyone the same opportunities is sufficient to enable them to have the same outcomes. Inclusion emphasises interdependence and presupposes that everyone is a part of society. Starting from this premise, society's institutions and practices should adapt to make this inclusion a reality.

The construction of people with learning disabilities as 'special' has, historically, been associated with offering them separate services, different from those of other children and adults in the community, with this, in turn, leading to restricted opportunities. On the other hand, the lack of priority given to the needs of people with learning disabilities has too often led to denying them access to appropriate services and supports, which, in turn, could mean they lack the most basic means of social participation. For example, if I need to be fed through a tube in my stomach, that fact should not, by itself, shape my life and mean that I cannot live at home, go to my local school or visit my local restaurant alongside my friends. However, if my life, health, and social participation depend on my tube feeding being appropriately monitored and my tube being inserted by someone who can do so safely, then I can only live safely when I have ready access to that support. Yet it is not necessarily the case that the best or safest way to develop, sustain, or deliver specialist support is in specialist settings, as the history of institutionalisation shows. Approaches such as intensive action show how the quality of life of people with profound and multiple disabilities depends on skills as much as setting (Nind and Hewett, 2001), but even appropriate approaches require investment in resources.

Thus, arguments about how best to include people with learning disabilities concern issues of philosophy and values, priorities, approach, and resources.

Critical review of practice

Models of participation

The literature on the involvement and participation of service users contains a number of schemas for categorising strategies to promote participation. These often suggest a hierarchy of interventions, with those that merely ask people for their opinions at the lower end of the scale and those that promote user control of services or policy at the top. These models have been developed primarily with references to the participation of service users. There is also significant literature on community development and community education, which has been used much more widely in community development and public health than in the field of disability (Freire, 1972). However, it also addresses the processes, both individual and collective, that can create liberation from oppression. Finally, the disability movement itself has a literature of personal and political struggle that stresses the vital importance of disabled people speaking for themselves, 'nothing about us, without us'.

It is recognised that there can be different approaches and levels of participation, so that, for example, people may have more or less control when becoming involved in designing their services or in policy consultations. Croft and Beresford (1996) argue for more serious participation that enables people to affect change rather than a raft of involvement strategies. In reviewing some of the range of opportunities that can be created for listening to people with learning disabilities, this chapter makes three assumptions. First, that being heard is essential to people with learning disabilities in view of their historic exclusion from having a voice and being in control. Second, that the social model of disability provides the framework within which approaches to participation can be critically reviewed. Third, that the debate about integration and inclusion suggests criteria against which such strategies could be evaluated. Is a particular approach being used in such a way as merely to reduce the perceived differences between the would-be participants and the 'norm' of participation? Or is the approach seeking to allow for diversity and actively to change the environment (be that of a public meeting, an individual's assessment or the way services are delivered) so that the participant can become a full and active agent?

Control over your own services

Within a consumer-based approach to services, making the individual service user, or someone acting in their interests, into the direct customer is one way to assert their control. In the UK, legislation now enables people who have been assessed as requiring services to receive direct funding rather than a pre-arranged package of care. Being in receipt of direct payments is one way of giving users greater control over the staff who work with them, and more flexibility in the way services are delivered to them. Both the English White Paper, *'Valuing People'* (Department of Health, 2001a) and *'The same as you?'* in Scotland (Scottish Executive, 2000), advocate direct payments for people with learning disabilities. Many local authority staff need more understanding of the possibilities and benefits of direct payments for people with learning disabilities (Beadle-Brown, 2002). In England, people with learning disabilities themselves reported on the obstacles to implementation (Department of Health, 2001b). The unequal access of people with learning disabilities to direct payments illustrates a fundamental principle for their social inclusion—that appropriate support is needed to ensure inclusion.

Simons (1999) has described how people can take a role in commissioning services. Within services delivered by provider agencies, there are a range of strategies being adopted to give service users greater control. These include enabling users to take part in the interviewing, selection, induction, and training of staff (Townley *et al*, undated). Bradley (2002) worked with self advocates from Quality Action Group in Stirling to produce training materials on communication for staff.

A further step towards greater control has been enabling individuals to have tenancies in their own name. The independent living movement stresses the significance of people being home owners or tenants in their own right, giving them a valued role in society through their position in the housing market (Pavilion, in collaboration with Advocacy in Action and the Notting Hill Housing Trust for the Joseph Rowntree Foundation, 1999). While legal status is an important marker of citizenship, it is important to stress that the priority for many individuals is 'a home of their own', the right to chose where and with whom they live, and the opportunity to move if they wish. Thus, the separation of housing and support brought about supported living is an important principle to ensure the rights of people with learning disabilities to live an ordinary life. A home of your own is not an aspiration only for people with low support needs. One of the pioneering initiatives in independent living in the UK was for two women with profound and multiple disabilities (Fitton *et al*, 1995).

Fundamental to enabling people to have control is support with decision-making. Values Into Action (VIA) have produced a guide to decision-making with people with high support needs, which explains how relationship and communication are central to effective support (Edge, 2001).

There are, at least, two stances underpinning developments towards greater control over services—consumerism and citizenship. Insofar as they lead to greater control and more freedom to exercise choice, both aspects may be important for the inclusion of people with learning disabilities, who have often not controlled their money or exercised many of the attributes of citizenship. However, considering citizenship from the perspective of empowering people with learning disabilities leads to an emphasis on the support that is needed to make social participation a reality. It is a model based in interdependence and mutuality.

Person-centred approaches

Person-centred approaches are a way of prioritising the person and his/her life, rather than the demands and contingencies of the service system. Person-centred planning is a family of techniques that have been developed to make the services and supports around an individual closer and more responsive to his/her real needs and wishes. The starting-point for person-centred planning is the dreams and aspirations of the individual and the strengths and opportunities that already exist in him/herself and in the people around him/her. The goal of person-centred planning is to put the person's life at the centre of the process and to challenge services and supports to respond to how that life could develop (Sanderson *et al*, 1997).

Person-centred approaches do not view the individual in isolation. Rather, they seek to identify, strengthen and enrich personal networks on the grounds that families and frie[illegible] the best guarantors of an individual's interests. This principle is at the root of the introduction of local area co-ordination into Scotland. Local Area Co-Ordination was developed in Western Australia (Disability Services Commission, 2001) and seeks to work in communities with individuals and families to link them into community supports so that they can live the life of their choosing in their community (Short Life Working Group, 2002).

Advocacy

Questions of power (who speaks?) and authenticity (with what authority?) are central to the development of advocacy by and for people with learning disabilities (Simons, 1995). The purpose of advocacy is to promote the interests of the individuals themselves. Self advocacy is when people speak on behalf of themselves or on behalf of others like themselves. People First is a self advocacy organisation, run by people with learning disabilities. In collective self advocacy, a group speaks up for their rights (People First Scotland, undated). Citizen advocacy, particularly important for people who cannot easily speak up for themselves, refers to representation of an individual's interests by an independent citizen. A citizen advocate is unpaid and, therefore, able to act independently on behalf of the person he/she represents. Citizen advocacy is based in long-term relationships between the advocate and his/her partner. Crisis advocacy is when an advocacy service is brought in to try to avoid a major abrogation of the person's rights; for example, if a discharge from hospital is being unnecessarily delayed.

Advocacy schemes may sometimes be funded by the agencies that an advocate may have to challenge. Solutions to this include the independent governance of the agency, standards, and codes of practice, and the protection of advocates through these routes. For example, in the Advocacy Project set up under *Valuing People,* the self advocacy work is managed by Values Into Action and the money to support citizen advocacy is being managed by the British Institute of Learning Disabilities. The greatest difficulty of advocacy schemes may not always be direct interference, but rather lack of response or resolution to the issues raised. There are good materials available about advocacy for people with learning disabilities themselves (for example, Loveman *et al*, 2001).

The criteria for good practice include whether the advocate is acting purely in the individual's interests and whether he/she is expressing that person's view or the best possible approximation to it. This may involve interpretation as well as communication support. The advocate is there to right the balance of power in favour of the individuals and to create a space in which their interests can be influential against all the other competing interests that may be present, including professional power, systems and practices, and resource constraints.

Voice and story

People with learning disabilities have, historically, suffered a double invisibility. They have been literally kept out of view, but also denied the means to comment on their story. This silencing is now being challenged in a variety of ways. The 'hidden histories' of people with learning disabilities, both in long-stay institutions and in the community, are being revealed by biographical and historical work with survivors (Atkinson *et al*, 1997; Atkinson and Williams, 1990). People are being encouraged to tell their own stories, stories of both extraordinary and ordinary lives (Atkinson *et al*, 2000; De Wit and Slater, Undated). Nor is this approach confined to history. Dan Goodley (2000) for example, has worked with self advocates to provide their own narratives of self-advocacy. In his book, individuals appear as activists who are part of a struggle for change.

There are at least two ways in which the expressive work of people with learning disabilities can challenge society to greater inclusion. One is to use a broader range of expressive media than the written word. People are using a variety of expressive media to tell their stories publicly, including: photography, video, theatre, and art (Goodley and Moore, 2002). The other is a question of content, challenging assumptions about what it is to be human and to live in society. Donna Williams, a woman with autism, has, in a series of books, asserted her difference and explained how she sees the world through different eyes (for example, Williams, 1999). Engagement with the expressive arts can also be a powerful tool for social inclusion, for it can demonstrate how intellectual access can be further improved (Lambe and Hogg, 2000). Grove and Park (2001) show how Shakespeare can be made accessible for people with profound disability.

Communication support

For people who have communication impairment in addition to their learning disability, access to communication support is extremely important to ensure that their wishes can be further taken into account. Without this access, it is likely that their life choices, even in small, everyday matters, may be extremely limited. David Goode (1994) pioneered the view that we can listen to those without speech. Training in augmentative and alternative communication can help practitioners find new ways to work with service users as communication partners. There are a number of resources available to help this learning. For example, the Augmentative and Alternative Communication Research Team at the University of Stirling has developed 'Talking Mats', a low tech system that uses picture symbols to help people think about topics so that they can then express their views and feelings more easily (Murphy and Cameron, undated). The same team have also produced resources that can be used in co-training users of communication systems, their communication partners, and speech and language therapists. Phoebe Caldwell has extended the range of approaches that can be used in communicating with people with profound and multiple impairment (Caldwell, 2002; Caldwell and Hoghton, 2000; Caldwell and Stevens, 1998). Total Communication strategies involve training the whole communication environment so that the individual's opportunities are maximised. Grove (2000) provides guidelines to help people understand communication by people with severe and profound learning disabilities.

The area of communication support illustrates a very important point about the social inclusion of people with learning disabilities. Few would argue that access to communication is a fundamental human right. Yet it is easy to overlook the fact that some people need support to be able to communicate, and to assume that those who do not speak cannot, in fact, make their wishes known. This is a misunderstanding that illustrates how the 'labelling' of people with learning disabilities can directly restrict their access to resources (people, knowledge and equipment, for example), which would enable their social inclusion.

Participatory research

Research can be seen as another arena in which effort has primarily been directed to making decisions about what happens to people with learning disabilities on their behalf, rather than with their active participation (Walmsley, 2001). The approach of participatory research seeks to give people with learning disabilities an active role in the design, conduct, and analysis of research that is relevant to them (Williams, 1999). For example, 'Real Choices' was a participatory action research project with young people about to leave school (Scottish Human Services Trust, 2002). Twelve young people from a class group in a special school in the Lothians, in Scotland, took part in the research, which used inclusive methods, such as physical games and drawings, to create discussion.

With support, people with learning disabilities have also conducted research and evaluated services (Whittaker, 1997). The Norah Fry Centre in Bristol worked alongside Swindon People First who obtained people's views of Direct Payments (Swindon People First/Norah Fry Research Centre, 2002). The Scottish Consortium for Learning Disability has plans to develop a network of 'research champions' who will contribute to round table discussions about research in Scotland, and act as mentors to researchers who want to make their work useful to people with learning disabilities (www.scld.org.uk)

Creating accessible information about research findings is another way that people with learning disabilities can use to become more active consumers of research and critical commentators on it. The 'Plain Facts' series is produced by the Norah Fry Centre at Bristol University and is 'a magazine about research for people with learning difficulties and their supporters'. It is produced on paper and on tape and uses pictures and clear language.

Changing public attitudes

Many people would agree with the force of social role valorisation theory that greater social participation by people with learning disabilities depends, in part, in their being perceived as valued and valuable citizens.

The workplace is a key arena where change in the attitudes of employers and other employees has the potential to directly affect the lives of people with learning disabilities by breaking down the barriers that prevent them entering the workforce. In Fife in Scotland, monies from the Change Fund, which were distributed to councils to enable them to implement change under 'The same as you?' review (SAY for short), have been used to develop a campaign to tell employers about the benefits of employing people with learning disabilities. The campaign, 'SAY, it's workable!' has been designed and is led by people with learning disabilities, working with the Fife employability team. They provide positive examples and information for people who may never have met someone with a learning disability before. As Jacqui, who introduces the information booklet that forms part of the campaign pack says, 'I want this campaign to change people's attitudes to people with learning disabilities. When they see us, they just see people with disabilities. I want them to see us as people—people who work' (Fife Council, 2002).

Participation in planning and policy implementation

Planners can give messages about who they think their plans are for, by the way that they produce their information. In Scotland, since the learning disability services review in 2000, local authorities and their partner agencies have had to produce joint strategic plans to indicate how they are going to bring about the changes recommended in the review. These plans are called Partnership in Practice Agreements (PiPs for short). North Lanarkshire Council chose to demonstrate an inclusive approach by producing the plan only in an accessible form in booklet and on video (North Lanarkshire Council, 2001). Called 'My Choice', the booklet uses photographs and symbols from the Boardmaker system to explain 'what has changed for some people with learning difficulties in North Lanarkshire.' It also says what change is still needed and how that will be done, including how the money will be used. Throughout, the stories of individuals are used to illustrate what the changes can mean for people's lives.

Conclusions

The issues reviewed here suggest a number of questions that policymakers, practitioners, researchers and students should consider when working in an inclusive way with an individual with learning disabilities. This final section spells out some of these issues and suggests questions that could be used as prompts by the reflective practitioner.

The quality and limits of personal relationships

The quality of the personal relationship between an individual and the practitioner is at the heart of inclusive practice. This focus on individuals and personal relationships can bring about a qualitative change in the environments in which people work, and many practitioners experience this as a direct benefit of working alongside people with learning disabilities. However, it is also essential to subject such practice to a critical review based on the analysis of power within those relationships and environments.

Being able to negotiate and constantly reinforce both the possibilities and the limits of the relationship is particularly important when working in individualised settings. For example, it is important that a worker is able to use his/her own capacities and interests as a tool for extending the individual's social inclusion. Workers may take the person to their home, introduce him/her to their family and friends and take him/her to their local pub. In doing so, they will need to be very clear with themselves, with their organisation and with the person they are working with what limits they will tolerate to this inclusion. Are they prepared for the person to visit them at any time, to marry their daughter, to get drunk in front of their neighbours? The reflective practitioner will constantly ask herself in whose interests she is acting and what the long-term implications are for the person she supports.

Power and immediacy

In the wish to involve people with learning disabilities in the public as well as the private sphere, it is possible to put people in the position where they are distanced from the issues that are of most immediate concern to them. Strategies to encourage participation need to remember that the personal is political and to allow space for individual experiences which can have a powerful and effective influence on the public debate. It is also very important not to lose sight of the practical realities of involvement for individuals. What other activities are they foregoing to take part in the public sphere? Are needs for transport and support being met? Without due consideration to these aspects, then exclusion will be promoted. What benefits accrue to the individual from his/her participation? This might be experience, training or money, but these need to be made real, rather than assuming that participation by itself is beneficial.

However, it would be disparaging to people with learning disabilities to suggest that they can only tell their personal stories. Without appropriate support, people can act as trustees, sit on national advisory groups and generally contribute to 'big picture' work.

The benefits of inclusive practice

General lessons can be learned from people with learning disabilities about how to change for the better the way everyday business is often conducted within organisations and public forums. For example, attending meetings, reviews or conferences that are run according to good practice guidelines for working with people with learning disabilities is likely to be a more personally rewarding experience for everyone involved. This is because everyone likes to feel heard, or have a chance to get it wrong and be able to be valued and contribute as an individual, in a setting in which there is space for direct personal interaction. This can, in turn, improve communication and decision-making.

Throughout this chapter, we have underlined a key message about the inclusion of people with learning disabilities. Inclusion cannot be an add-on. It demands a revision of how independence and citizenship are understood. These do not mean that you can only have rights if you can do things on your own. Rather, support across a wide range of areas of life, communication, intellectual access, and social participation, for example, is a requirement to ensure the social participation of all citizens. Without such participation, society as a whole is deprived of the contributions and talents of people with learning disabilities.

References

Atkinson D *et al* (2000) *Good Times, Bad Times: Women with Learning Difficulties Telling their Stories*. BILD, Kidderminster

Atkinson D, Jackson M, Walmsley J (1997) *Forgotten Lives: Exploring the History of Learning Disability*. BILD, Kidderminster

Atkinson D, Williams F (1990) *Know Me As I Am*. Hodder and Stoughton/Open University, London

Beadle-Brown J (2002) Direct payments for people with severe learning disabilities: a service case study and implications for policy. *Tizard Learn Disabil Rev* **74**: 10–16

Bradley A (2002) *Positive Approaches to Communication: A Workbook to Support the Mandatory Units of the Certificates in Working with People who have Learning Disabilities*. BILD, Kidderminster

Caldwell P (2002) *Learning the Language: Video-Based resource on building relationships with people with severe learning disability, autistic spectrum disorder and challenging behaviours*. Pavilion Publishing, Brighton

Caldwell P, Hoghton, M (2000) *You Don't Know What It's Like*. Pavilion Publishing, Brighton

Caldwell P, Stevens P (1998) *Person To Person: Establishing contact and communication with people with profound disabilities or with those whose behaviour is challenging*. Pavilion Publishing, Brighton

Campbell J, Oliver M (1996) *Disability Politics: Understanding our Past, Changing our Future*. Routledge, London

Croft S, Beresford P (1996) The politics of participation. In: Taylor D, ed. *Critical Social Policy: A Reader.* Sage, London

Curtice L (2001) The social and spiritual inclusion of people with learning disabilities: a liberating challenge? *Contact* **136**: 15–23

Department of Health (2001a) *Valuing People: A New Strategy for Learning Disability for the 21st Century.* HMSO, London

Department of Health (2001b)*Nothing About Us Without Us.* Department of Health, London

De Wit M, Slater D (undated) *Rediscovering Ourselves: Assisting People with Learning Disabilities to Rediscover their Personal History.* Pavilion Publishing, Brighton

Disability Services Commission (2001) *Local Area Co-Ordination Framework.* Disability Services Commission, Perth

Edge J (2001) *Who's in Control? Decision-making by People with Learning Difficulties who have High Support Needs.* Values Into Action, London

Fife Council (2002) *SAY, It's Workable: Celebrating Diversity in the Workplace.* Fife Council, Glenrothes

Fitton P, O'Brien C, Wilson J (1995) *Home at Last: How Two Young Women with Profound Intellectual and Multiple Disabilities Achieved their Own Home.* Jessica Kingsley, London

Freire P (1972) *Pedagogy of the Oppressed.* Penguin Books, Middlesex

Goode D (1994) *A World Without Words: The Social Construction of Children Born Deaf and Blind.* Temple University Press, Philadelphia

Goodley D (2001) Learning difficulties: the social model of disability and impairment: challenging epistemologies. *Disabil Soc* **16**(2): 207–31

Goodley D (2000) *Self-Advocacy in the Lives of People with Learning Difficulties: The Politics of Resilience.* Open University Press, Buckingham

Goodley D, Moore M (2002) *Disability Arts Against Exclusion.* BILD, Kidderminster

Grove N (2000) *See What I Mean: Guidelines to Aid Understanding of Communication by People with Severe and Profound Learning Disabilities.* BILD/Mencap, Kidderminster

Grove N, Park K (2001) *Social Cognition through Drama and Literature for People with Learning Disabilities—Macbeth in Mind.* Jessica Kingsley Publishers, London

King's Fund Centre (1980) *An Ordinary Life.* King's Fund Centre, London

Lambe L, Hogg J (2000) *Creative Arts and People with Profound and Multiple Learning Disabilities: Innovative Practices to Broaden the Experiences of People with Profound and Multiple Learning Disabilities.* Pavilion Publishing, Brighton

Loveman L, England P, Unstead N (2001) *Advocacy Workbook for People with Learning Difficulties.* BILD, Kidderminster

Murphy J, Cameron L (undated) *Talking Mats and Learning Disability,* a training package. AAC Research Team, University of Stirling, Stirling

Nind M, Hewett D (2001) *A Practical Guide to Intensive Interaction.* BILD, Kidderminster

North Lanarkshire Council (2001) *My Choice: Partnership in Practice Agreement 2001.* North Lanarkshire Council Social Work Department, Motherwell

Pavilion in Collaboration with Advocacy in Action and the Notting Hill Housing Trust for the Joseph Rowntree Foundation (1999) *This Is My Home: Challenging the Language of Care and Control.* Pavilion Publishing, Brighton

People First Scotland (undated) *Self-Advocacy.* http://www.firstscotland.fsnet.co.uk

Priestley M (1998) Constructions and creations: idealism, materialism and disability theory. *Disabil Society* **13**(1): 75–94

Sanderson H, Jennedy J, Ritchie P, Goodwin G (1997) *People, Plans and Possibilities.* Scottish Human Services, Edinburgh

Scottish Executive (2000) *The Same as You? Review of Services for People with Learning Disabilities in Scotland.* The Stationery Office, Edinburgh

SHS Trust (2002) *Real Choices: A Participatory Action Research Project involving Young People with Learning Difficulties who are about to Leave School.* Scottish Human Services Trust, Edinburgh

Short Life Working Group on Local Area Co-Ordination (2002) *Recommendations to the National Implementation Group.* www.scld.org.uk

Simons K (1999) *A Place at the Table? Involving People with Learning Difficulties in Purchasing and Commissioning Services.* BILD, Kidderminster

Simons K (1995) Empowerment and advocacy. In: Malin N, ed. *Services for People with Learning Disabilities.* Routledge, London

Swain J, Finkelstein V, French S, Oliver M, eds (1993) *Disabling Barriers—Enabling Environments.* Sage, London

Swindon People First/Norah Fry Research Centre (2002) *Journey to Independence: What Self Advocates tell us about Direct Payments.* BILD, Kidderminster

Thomas C (1999) *Female Forms: Experiencing and Understanding Disability.* Open University Press, Buckingham

Townley R *et al* (undated) *Getting Involved in Choosing Staff: A practical guide to successfully involving people with learning disabilities in choosing staff to work in their services.* Pavilion Publishing in association with the Norah Fry Research Centre and the Joseph Rowntree Foundation, Brighton

Walmsley J (2001) Normalisation, emancipatory research and inclusive research in learning disability. *Disabil Society* **16**(2): 187–205

Whittaker A (1997) *Looking at Our Services—Service Evaluation by People with Learning Difficulties.* King's Fund Centre, London

Williams D (1999) *Like Colour to the Blind: Soul Searching and Soul Finding.* Jessica Kingsley, London

Williams V (1999) Researching together. *Br J Learn Disabil* **27**: 48–51

Wolfensberger W (1983) Social role valorization: a proposed new term for the principle of normalisation. *Mental Retard* **21**: 234–39

4 Integration: Developing quality and standards

Margaret Whoriskey

Introduction

Quality and standards are now commonly used terms underpinning national policy across health and social care services, as evidenced in recent publications (Department of Health, 1998; Scottish Executive, 2002; 2000a; 2000b; 1999; 1998). A 'First Class Service—Quality in the NHS' was published in 1998 and provides the framework for quality and clinical governance for the NHS in England and Wales. In Scotland, 'Our National Health, A Plan for Action, a Plan for Change' (Scottish Executive, 2000b) emphasises the need for clear national clinical and services standards and robust quality monitoring arrangements for all NHS services. Similarly, Aiming for Excellence (Scottish Executive, 1999) sets out the policy for the regulation of social work services and the framework for the development of national care standards. While these national policy directives relate to the broad range of health and social care services, they are wholly relevant for services to people with learning disabilities.

In the area of learning disabilities, the focus on quality and standards is not new. There have been many attempts over the years to develop appropriate quality measures to monitor the quality of care and quality of life of people with learning disabilities who use services. Involving people, who use the service, and their family carers, in this area is essential, but can be neglected. This chapter will address the historical context of quality and standards, and developing focus on 'quality of life' measures within learning disability services; examine some current approaches to quality monitoring in the UK, and identify how users and carers should be involved in promoting integrated care.

Historical context

The focus on quality and standards within learning disability services was prompted by a number of enquiries and reports that identified poor conditions within some learning disability and psychiatric institutions in the UK and elsewhere. The description of the 'back ward' by Jones (1960) painted a grim picture of overcrowding, neglect and, in some cases, outright brutality.

Reports of enquiries set up to investigate allegations of ill-treatment became a feature of social policy literature during the 1960s and 1970s (e.g. Ely Hospital: DHSS, 1969; Normansfield: DHSS, 1978). They presented a catalogue of failure at all levels of service provision and service management (Martin, 1984).

In his analysis of reports by committees of enquiry into 19 hospitals, Martin cites common features found in these hospitals that more or less mirrored the studies of hospitals in the 1950s (e.g. Barton, 1959; NCCL, 1951). These included: geographical and professional isolation; abandonment of patients by their community; lack of support towards staff; failure of leadership among all professional groups, and 'corruption of care'.

Such issues contributed to the establishment of the Hospital Advisory Service in England and Wales and the Scottish Hospital Advisory Service (SHAS) in Scotland in 1970, to provide 'independent' monitoring of services to vulnerable groups, including people with learning disabilities.

An important development, which influenced the quality agenda in the field of learning disabilities, was the 'Normalisation Principle ' (Wolfensberger, 1972). It has proved to be an influential concept in debates concerning the most appropriate way of providing services for people with learning disabilities in Scandinavia, North America, and the UK. This influence has broadened to include other disability groups. Normalisation offered a theoretical model from which to develop good practice. In particular, it offered a way of conceptualising the pull towards negative practice and an important model of how to reverse this. A series of evaluation materials and approaches were developed known as PASS (Program Analysis of Service Systems) and PASSING (Program Analysis of Services Systems' Implementing of Normalizing Goals) whose primary use lies in assessing the extent to which services implement the principle of Normalisation (Wolfensberger and Glenn, 1975; Wolfensberger and Thomas, 1983). Such approaches were adopted by many residential and day services in the UK during the 1980s, although they are less evident today.

A range of quality measures has been developed for learning disability services in the UK and elsewhere and some attempts made to put in place measurable standards. In the late 1970s, the National Development Group (NDG) for Mentally Handicapped[1]. People was asked by the then Secretary of State for Social Services to suggest their own checklist of the criteria for a good mental handicap service. The NDG was of the view that there is considerable agreement on most of the basic principles on which services should be based, as identified in the Jay Committee Report (DHSS, 1979). In 1980, the National Development Group produced the checklist of standards (NDG, 1980), which incorporated measures of the physical environment, opportunities for individual development, and the provision of appropriate services. The standards were set by 'interested' experts based on, what informal opinion believed should be, the basic principles reflected by services in their quality. A number of checklists and monitoring instruments were drawn on in the development of these standards (e.g. King *et al*, 1971; Raynes *et al*, 1979). The authors stated that the completion of the checklist would provide a range of detailed information on the basis of which the quality of a local service could be evaluated and plans made for improvements. Despite the development of such standards, there has not been wide spread adoption of this approach

1 Mental Handicap was terminology used at that time

within services. However, the developing focus on standards and their measurement has led to attention being given to quality of life as a key issue for services to address.

A major influence on the quality agenda has been John O'Brien's (1987) formulation of the five service accomplishments which draw on the implications of normalisation in terms of what services should try to achieve or accomplish for users. The five accomplishments focus on:

- Ensuring community presence
- Supporting choices
- Developing competencies and skills
- Enhancing respect
- Ensuring participation.

They place major emphasis upon delineating the implications of normalisation, in terms of the lifestyle or quality of life of members of devalued groups, and return choice to a central position in normalisation. Many services have striven to adopt these principles and some researchers and service providers consider these areas in the context of service evaluation and quality monitoring.

Quality of life

Quality of life has a central position in the evaluation of services for people with learning disabilities, due to the major role services play in contributing to, or even determining, individual lifestyles (Felce and Perry, 1995). Reasons include:

- Greater general social awareness about issues of quality
- Growing concern about quality of life in community placements for people with learning disabilities
- Dissatisfaction with current approaches to monitoring and evaluating services outcomes and quality of service
- Wider acceptance of user viewpoints in determining satisfaction

- Some acceptance of quality of life as a concept guiding clinical decision-making and social and health policy formation.

In the area of learning disabilities, evaluation of quality of life has been fundamental to many publications on how services should be delivered. In the 1970s and 80s, quality of life evaluations frequently focussed on three aspects:

- Quality of the physical environment in which people live (e.g. King *et al*, 1971)
- Quality of care people receive from staff who look after them (e.g. Hemming *et al*, 1981)
- Degree of integration into neighbourhood as measured by use of physical facilities (e.g. Butler and Bjannes, 1978).

Over recent years, a number of areas concerned with quality of life have received attention in evaluation studies on services for people with learning disabilities (Emerson and Hatton, 1994; Hatton and Emerson, 1996). In particular, objective indicators, such as individuals' skills and competencies, living environments, health, social care and engagement in activities, have received attention. However, the more subjective areas, such as emotional well-being and personal satisfaction with lifestyle, while well reported in the general literature on quality of life, appear to be relatively neglected in the area of learning disabilities. Authors, such as Felce and Perry (1995), emphasise the need to incorporate both subjective and objective measures of quality of life.

Quality of life measures specific to the area of learning disabilities are emerging, as the role of hospital closures, community integration, social inclusion and mainstreaming call for an outcome indicator sensitive enough for the evaluation of the shift in provision of services.

Current approaches to measuring quality

There is a range of approaches that aim to address both internal and external quality monitoring across health and social care services. For ease of reference, these are grouped under three headings—Internal Standards and Systems, External Optional Audits/Inspections, and Mandatory or Statutory Standards and Inspection.

Internal standards and systems

Services, in general, will operate some internal quality monitoring, which include compliance with specific standards and measures. NHS boards and trusts have structures in place to address quality monitoring within the context of clinical governance. Local authorities and service providers will also address quality monitoring in relation to the commissioning and provision of services. Services may operate quality groups or quality circles to share good practice and identify areas requiring action. Audit and research contribute to a quality approach, although such activity can be viewed as optional. Increasingly, attention is being paid to quality of life measures for people using learning disability services.

External optional audits/ inspections

Across the UK, there are many examples of standards and quality audits which, although optional, are viewed as desirable. Some tools in use are generic and relevant to a wide range of services, whereas others are specific to conditions or care groups. Such approaches may lead to accreditation in certain areas and provide an external validation of service quality. Examples include Investors in People (IIP), Kings Fund Accreditation and Charter Mark awards. Within the field of learning disability, the Quality Network provides a user focussed evaluation of service quality and such an approach is now being used in Scotland across health and social care services. The evaluation has a focus on outcomes and continuous improvement, and includes a self review by service providers, together with external validation.

Mandatory or statutory standards and inspection

Services are required to meet certain standards in order to comply with regulations and policy. This will include areas, such as health and safety.

There are currently a number of organisations across the UK responsible for setting and inspecting standards and promoting quality improvement. The situation in Scotland differs somewhat to the rest of the UK in relation to the role and responsibilities of different bodies and inspection methodology. The main organisations are referred to below with brief descriptions of current areas of responsibility.

In England and Wales, the **Health Advisory Service** (**HAS**) and, in Scotland, the **Scottish Health Advisory Service** (**SHAS**) were established as independent bodies in 1970, with authority to carry out mandatory visits to health services to review the quality of these services for vulnerable people in long stay hospitals. HAS became an independent charity and was established by the Department of Health in 1997 to work in mental health and older people services only. In England and Wales, there is currently no specific external inspection of NHS services for people with learning disabilities.

SHAS is an independent public sector organisation accountable to the First Minister. Since 1970, SHAS has continued its role in relation to 'peer review' of services for people with learning or physical disabilities, people with mental illness and older people, with increasing emphasis on community-based services. SHAS has developed quality indicators/standards (SHAS, 2000b) for evaluating community and in-patient health services for children and adults with learning disabilities and the other care groups. This is referred to further below.

The **Clinical Standards Board for Scotland** (**CSBS**) was established in 1999 to ensure the NHS Scotland delivers the highest possible standard of care. The key function of the CSBS is to promote public confidence in NHS Scotland by driving forward and improving standards. A process of accreditation based on a system of peer review is used to evaluate performance of NHS service providers. Written standards, designed to assess the quality of an activity, service or organisation, guide the process. While there are no standards specific to learning disability services at present, many of the standards have a general applicability to health service provision. The generic standards (CSBS, 2002) underpin all services to ensure patients receive safe and effective treatment, that services respond to patients' needs and preferences, and that people are involved in decisions about their care. Condition specific standards are being developed, which relate to the actual delivery of care and treatment for particular illnesses, for example coronary heart disease (CSBS, 2000) and schizophrenia (CSBS, 2001) and these areas are as relevant to people with learning disabilities as to any one else.

A new specialist health board was established in Scotland in January 2003, called **NHS Quality Improvement Scotland**. The current work of SHAS, the CSBS and other organisations, such as the **Health Technology Board for Scotland**, will be integrated within this new organisation. NHS Quality Improvement Scotland will be charged with the development of a national strategy for improving the quality of patient care and with co-ordinating the work of Scotland's clinical effectiveness organisations.

In England and Wales, a C**ommission for Health Improvement** (**CHI**) was established in 1999 to improve the quality of patient care in the NHS. It does this by reviewing the care provided by the NHS and aims to address unacceptable variations in NHS patient care by identifying good practice, and areas where care could be improved. Like the CSBS, CHI conducts clinical governance reviews in all NHS organisations on a continuous programme. Specific studies are also carried out based on the recommendations of National Service Frameworks (NSF). NSFs are developed by the Department of Health in England, and the Welsh Assembly Government in Wales to set standards that will achieve greater consistence in the availability and quality of services for a range of major care areas and disease groups. NSFs make recommendations about the quality of service that patients should expect from a specific area of health care. A cancer care study was completed in 2001 (CHI,

2001) and further studies by CHI and the Audit Commission are underway, or planned, in coronary heart disease, older people, and mental health.

In Scotland during 2000 and 2002, Scottish ministers set up the National Care Standards Committee (NCSC) to develop national standards; for example, for people in receipt of residential day care and care at home services. There are specific care standards for people with learning disabilities who are resident in care homes (Scottish Executive, 2001). These were developed from the point of view of people who use services. They describe what each individual person can expect from the service provider and focus on the quality of life that the person using the service actually experiences. The **Care Commission in Scotland** was established in April 2002 and has responsibility to register and inspect all non-NHS providers of care, including local authorities. Similar arrangements also exist in England and Wales with the setting up of **The National Care Standards Commission** in April 2002 to regulate social care and private and voluntary health services

Most external inspection bodies are concerned with service issues. However, there is also a need to ensure quality of care and welfare from an individual standpoint. The **Mental Welfare Commission for Scotland** (MWC) has a statutory duty, under the Mental Health (Scotland) Act 1984, to protect people who are vulnerable because of mental illness or learning disability, who may not be receiving proper care, be unfairly treated, and who may be exploited. This duty includes people in hospital, in local authority, voluntary run or private accommodation, or in their own house. The Commission also has new responsibilities under the Adults with Incapacity (Scotland) 2000. The MWC has statutory responsibilities to visit all learning disability and psychiatric hospitals on an annual basis and, increasingly, has been visiting people with learning disabilities who live in the community. The MWC has a duty to make enquiry into any case where it appears there may be ill-treatment or deficiency in care or treatment, or damage or loss to property for any person with a learning disability or mental illness. Some recent enquiries have focussed on individuals with learning disabilities (Mental Welfare Commission, 2000; 2001) and standards of care and treatment. In England and Wales, **The Mental Health Act Commission** has a much more restrictive role, which is mainly concerned with patients who are detained under the Act.

SHASA: Qualitative approach

As noted above, there are a number different organisations charged with the development and monitoring of standards for health and social care services. In Scotland, the new NHS Quality Improvement Special Health Board will provide an overall structure for external quality monitoring within the NHS and will incorporate the current work undertaken by SHAS. Since 1970, SHAS has undertaken independent reviews of health services for people with learning disabilities and other vulnerable care groups. Review teams are drawn from a network of more than 200 people in health service, social work, voluntary organisations, lay people and users and carers. In May 2000, Learning Disability Quality Indicators were published. Quality indicators were developed to ensure SHAS, as a quality driven organisation, is consistent in its approach to inspecting and advising on the planning and provision of health care in Scotland. The quality indicators were developed by considering the research available in the area of quality monitoring in learning disability services (e.g. Emerson and Hatton, 1998; Felce and Emerson, 1996; Hatton *et al*, 1999; Lanconi *et al*, 1996; Whoriskey, 1998) and relevant guidance and policy (e.g. Department of Health, 1995; 1999a; 1999b). The views of people who use services and staff from health and social work service were involved in their development. The quality indicators serve as agreed descriptions of best practice and current policy. A service user version (SHAS, 2000a) and Symbol Version (SHAS, 2001a) of the quality indicators are available to record direct experiences from service users and carers. At present, there are seven key quality indicators, although these are currently being reviewed to take account of policy development, organisational changes within the NHS and the integration of SHAS with NHS Quality Improvement Scotland. The quality indicators topic areas are summarised in *Table 4.1* below. *Table 4.2* provides an example of specific quality indicators.

Table 4.1: Summary—SHAS learning disability quality indicators

	Topic	Principle
1.	Planning and assessing need	A needs assessment is undertaken, which informs the strategic direction for the service
2.	Delivery of health care: • Health promotion • Meeting general health needs • Transition from child to adult services • Meeting specialist health needs	Service users have access to general and specialised health care services, based on their identified health needs
3.	Service users' involvement • Planning and assessment • Access to health records • Complaints	Services users are actively involved in the planning and delivery of services
4.	Joint working	There are clear and agreed arrangements and identified roles within organisations to ensure joint working is taken forward
5.	Environment (inpatient services) • Safety • Access • Privacy and personalisation • Social, recreational and day opportunities	Service users are supported in an internal and external environment that is compatible with safety, security, privacy, dignity, freedom from exploitation and overall well-being
6.	Advocacy services	All service users should have access to an independent advocate, and services should be able to show how the advocacy process is integrated into the operation of the service
7.	Clinical governance	The trust has corporate accountability for clinical performance

Table 4.2: Quality indicator 2: Delivery of healthcare

Principle: Service users have access to general and specialised health care services, based on their identified health needs

	Quality indicator statement		Evaluation criteria	How to assess
2.1	There is local information on all service users' needs to support planning and service delivery	2.1.1 2.1.2	Confidentiality of data and protection procedures in place Information is available and up-to-date	Review information Discuss with variety of staff in all agencies Discuss with users and carers
2.2	People accessing health services have an up-to-date multidisciplinary care plan	2.2.1 2.2.2 2.2.3	There are care plans in place There is evidence of service user and relative and/or advocates involvement There is evidence of efforts to take account of any special communication needs	Review care plans and their management with community teams and provider services Discuss with staff, GPs, users and relatives
	Health promotion			
2.3	The trust has agreed policy on health education and promotion activies, including sexual health	2.3.1 2.3.2	There is a health education policy in place which ensures: • educational materials are available and utilised • staff training programmes are in place • involvement of health education departments There is evidence of interagency agreement/working	Review health education policy and information provision See educational materials used

SHAS assessment framework

The assessment framework has been designed to measure how well a service is meeting the SHAS quality indicators. This involves NHS trusts and boards in association with local authorities completing a self-assessment. SHAS then undertakes a parallel assessment, using the same tool, with the right to visit any part of the services over three to four days. SHAS continues to keep an organisational overview and considers services in the context of the broader organisation and inter-agency working. For learning disability services, SHAS expects involvement from children and adult services, alongside primary care, acute hospitals, and a specialised learning disability service. There is a strong interface with social care services and SHAS welcomes the opportunity to visit users in a range of residential and day settings, and in their own home. The assessment framework provides ratings from strongly disagree to strongly agree. For ease of reference, the criteria are outlined below:

Strongly agree	The statement represents a completely accurate description of what is happening and is an example of good practice
Agree	On balance, the quality indicator is being met in a satisfactory manner
Disagree	There are significant gaps in meeting the quality indicator and work needs to be done to improve things
Strongly disagree	The quality indicator is not being met at all
Not relevant	The statement does not apply in this setting
Don't know	When there is insufficient information to answer the question

The response categories are there to give guidance and are not a scoring mechanism. *Table 4.3* provides an example of a completed (fictional) assessment framework statement.

Table 4.3: SHAS Assessment Framework (Quality Indicator 2.5 and 2.6)

		Strongly disagree	Disagree	Agree	Strongly agree	Not relevant	Don't know
Meeting general health needs							
2.5	The primary care team/LHCC knows how many people with a learning disability are registered with their practice						
2.5.1	Appropriate information is recorded on needs		X	X*			
2.5.2	LHCC/Practices have a register	X					
Commentary There is no systematic information systems in place and trusts are awaiting further guidance from the Scottish Executive on the development of data bases in line with SAY recommendation. The National Special Needs Data Base for children is in place and information on children with special needs is recorded and generally known to GPs							
2.6	There is a named nurse for each GP Practice						
2.6.1	Every GP practice has access to a named learning disability nurse, who is able to facilitate access to primary and specialist services as appropriate and provide support to other members of the health care team			X*	X		
Commentary There are named learning disability staff identified for GP practices and this has assisted in greater awareness of the needs of people with learning disabilities. Community learning disability nurses are now based within LHCCs and professional support is provided from learning disability services. Some innovative training sessions have been arranged for primary care staff and clear referral protocols are in place. For children with learning disabilities, specialist health visitor posts provide support to the primary care team							

X* children's services
X adult services

SHAS reports are public and provide a narrative overview and description of the service. In addition, there is a detailed account of the review team's findings against the Quality Indicators matrix. Examples of good practice are also identified, along with specific recommendations for improvement.

Role of users and carers

One of the major difficulties in the evaluation of services for people with learning disabilities is that some clients of the services are neither able to express their own views, nor are they given the opportunity to identify desired outcomes for services they receive. There is a general consensus that the opinion of the users of services should be sought.

While it has been long recognised that people should be involved in assessing their 'quality of life', many researchers excluded the view of people with a learning disability on the basis that they are least able to conceptualise and articulate and, therefore, focus on the more objective measures. In 1981, Landesman-Dwyer, in an address to the Residents Committee on Mental Retardation in the US, stated, 'As much as possible, assessment of quality life should be from the viewpoint of individual clients¼rather than our own perspective'. A number of researchers have shown that, with care, it is now practical to involve these individuals in research and service evaluation (e.g. Cullen *et al*, 1995; Flynn, 1989; Lowe and dePaiva, 1990; McKenzie, 1990; Walker *et al*, 1993).

As a contribution to this aim, SHAS, along with users and family carers, has developed User and Symbol Versions of the Learning Disability Quality Indicators (SHAS, 2000a and b; 2001a) to assist in gaining views directly from users and carers about their experiences of health services. Examples of these are shown below. Services are required to consult with users and carers and collate information on responses as part of a self-assessment. SHAS then carries out a visit to the service and meets directly with users and carers. This feedback is crucial to the service inspection and views of users and carers are covered at the beginning of the report.

SHAS Learning Disability Quality Indicators—User Version

Topic: How do you get your Health Care

QUESTIONS

(11) Have you had any problems getting appointments

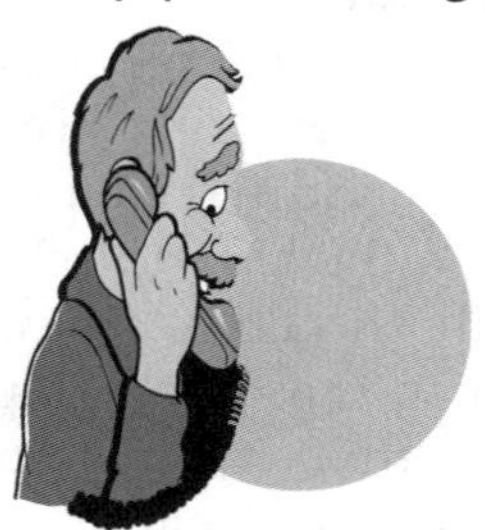

(12) Have you had any other problems?

What happened?

(13) Have you been to a hospital recently?

Did someone tell you what was going to happen?

Were you given information before you went to hospital?

Was someone you know able to stay with you?

SHAS Learning Disability Quality Indicators: Symbol Version

(6) Do you know about being healthy?

yes
no
Do you know who to ask?
yes
no

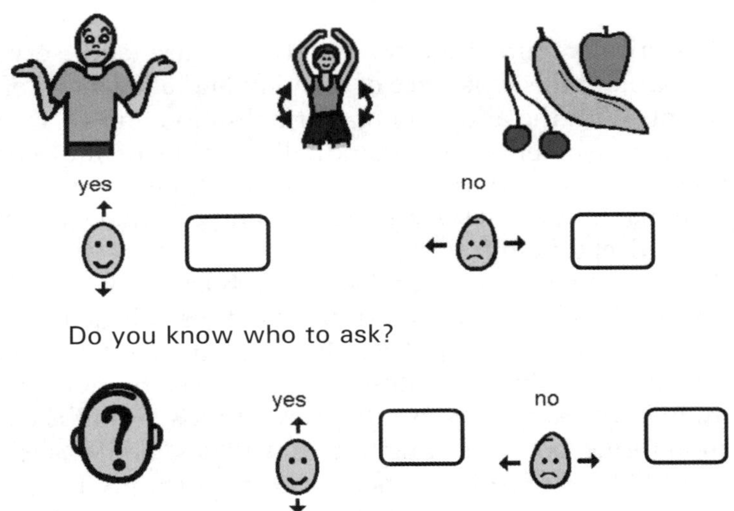

What is good?

What could be better?

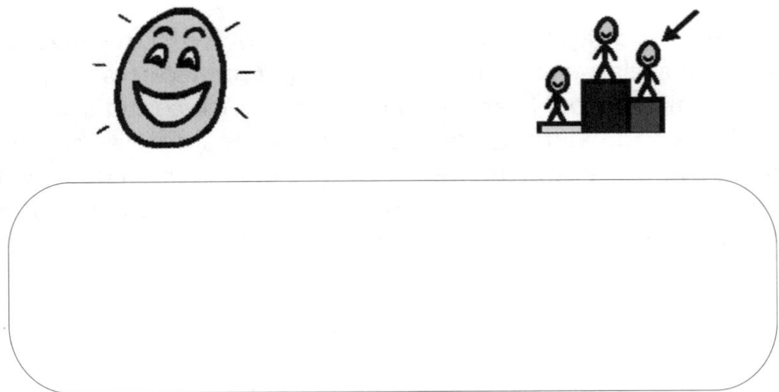

The Quality Network also provides a good example of user involvement in service evaluation.

Conclusion

Historically, attention to quality of care and services centred around the avoidance of scandals and allegations of ill-treatment. With the adoption of Normalisation and O' Brien's five accomplishments, an individual's quality of life, which includes care and services, is the outcome of choice in service evaluations. Internal service standards and external standards need to reflect this shift.

We can be reassured that there are robust quality monitoring systems in place with new arrangements established in Scotland and elsewhere in the UK. However, it may be of some concern that learning disability health services do not receive attention in the same way as other care groups, from the external monitoring bodies in England and Wales, bodies such as CHI and HAS. In Scotland, there is an opportunity to ensure that services for people with learning disabilities retain an important focus within NHS Quality Improvement Scotland and that the needs of people with learning disabilities are appropriately considered in the development of other standards. The interface between health and social care systems needs to be addressed by taking forward an integrated approach to service quality.

Users and carers must be centrally involved in the development of standards and quality monitoring for services of which they are in receipt. There is a need for service commissioners, providers and external monitoring bodies to address this, as a priority issue central to the government 'Patient and Public Involvement' initiative. The validity of service evaluation must be called into question if this is not realised.

References

Barton R (1959) *Institutional Neurosis*. John Wright, Bristol

Butler E, Bjannes AT (1978). Activities and the use of time by retarded persons in community care facilities. In: Sackett GP ed. *Observing Behaviour*, Vol. 1. University Park Press, London

Clinical Standards Board For Scotland (2002) Clinical Standards—Generic Standards. CSBS, Scotland

Clinical Standards Board for Scotland (2001) *Clinical Standards—Schizophrenia*. CSBS, Scotland

Clinical Standards Board for Scotland (2000) *Clinical Standards—Secondary Prevention Following Myocardial Infarction*. CSBS, Scotland

Commission for Health Improvement (2001) *Review of Cancer Services*. CHI, Scotland

Cullen C, Whoriskey M, Mackenzie K, *et al* (1995) The effects of deinstitutionalisation on adults with learning disabilities. *J Intellect Disabil Res* **39**: 484–94

Department of Health (1999a) *Signposts for Success— Commissioning and Providing Health Services for People with Learning Disabilities*. HMSO, London

Department of Health (1999b) *Once a Day—Primary Care Services for People with Learning Disabilities*. HMSO, London

Department of Health (1998) *A First Class Service—Quality in the NHS*. HMSO, London

Department of Health (1995) *The Health of the Nation: A Strategy for People with Learning Disabilities*. HMSO, London

Department of Health and Social Security (1979) *Report of the Committee of Enquiry into Mental Handicap Nursing and Care (The Jay Report)*. HMSO, London

Department of Health and Social Security (1978) *Normansfield Enquiry*. HMSO, London

Department of Health and Social Security (1969). *Report of the Committee of Injury into Allegations of Ill Treatment of Patients and other Irregularities at the Ely Hospital, Cardiff*. HMSO, London

Emerson E, Hatton C (1998) Residential provision for people with intellectual disabilities in England, Wales and Scotland. *J App Res Intellect Disabil* **11**: 1–14

Emerson E, Hatton C (1994) *Moving Out—Relocation from Hospital to Community*. HMSO, London

Felce D, Perry J (1995) Quality of life. It's definitions and measurement. *Res Development Disabil* **16**: 51–57

Flynn M (1989) *Independent Living for Adults with Mental Handicap. 'A Place of My Own'*. Cassell, London

Hatton C, Emerson E (1996) *Residential Provision for People with Learning Disabilities: A Research Review*. Hester Adrian Research Centre, University of Manchester, Manchester

Hatton C, Rivers M, Mason H, *et al* (1999) Organisational culture and staff outcomes in services for people with intellectual disabilities. *J Intellect Disabil Res* **43**: 206–18

Hemming H, Lavender T, Pill R (1981) Quality of life of mentally retarded adults transferred from large institutions to new small units. *Am J Ment Defic* **86**: 157–69

Jones K (1960) *Mental Health and Social Policy: 1845–1959*. Routledge and Kegan Paul, London

King R, Raynes N, Tizard J (1971) *Patterns of Residential Care*. Routledge and Kegan Paul, London

Lanconi GE, O'Reilly MF, Emerson E (1996) A review of choice research with people with severe and profound developmental disabilities. *Res Development Disabil* **17**: 391–411

McKenzie K (1990). Quality of life of mentally handicapped people: A pilot study. M Phil thesis unpublished. University of Edinburgh

Martin J (1984) *Hospitals in Trouble*. Blackwell, Oxford

Mental Welfare Commission For Scotland (2001) *Deficiency in Care and Treatment—Inquiry into the Care and Treatment of Mr B. Annual Report 2000–2001*. Mental Welfare Commission for Scotland, Edinburgh

Mental Welfare Commission for Scotland (1999) *Deficiency in Care and Treatment Inquiry—Ms P. Annual Report 1998–1999*. Mental Wellfare Commission for Scotland, Edinburgh

National Development Group (1980). *Improving the Quality of Services for Mentally Handicapped People: A Checklist of Standards*. Department of Health and Social Security, London

National Council For Civil Liberties (NCCL) (1951) *Community Care Development*. HMSO, London

O'Brien J (1987) A guide to lifestyle planning: using the activities catalogue to integrate services and natural support systems. In: Wilcox BW, Bellamy GT, eds. *The Activities Catalogue: An Alternative Curriculum for Youth and Adults with Severe Disabilities*. Brookes, Baltimore

Raynes NV, Pratt MW, Roses S (1979) *Organisational Structure and the Care of the Mentally Handicapped*. Croom Helm, London

Scottish Health Advisory Service (2001a) *Learning Disability Quality Indicators—Symbol Version*. Scottish Health Advisory Service, Edinburgh

Scottish Health Advisory Service (2001b) *Learning Disability—Assessment Framework*. Scottish Health Advisory Service, Edinburgh

Scottish Health Advisory Service (2000a) *Learning Disability Quality Indicators—User Version*.Scottish Health Advisory Service, Edinburgh

Scottish Health Advisory Service (2000b) *Learning Disability Quality Indicators*. Scottish Health Advisory Service, Edinburgh

Scottish Executive (2002) *Promoting Health, Supporting Inclusion—The National Review of the Contribution of all Nurses and Midwives to the Care and Support of People with Learning Disabilities*. The Stationery Office, Edinburgh

Scottish Executive (2001) *National Care Standard: Care Homes for People with Learning Disabilities*. The Stationery Office, Edinburgh??

Scottish Executive (2000) *Our National Health—A Plan for Action, a Plan for Change*. The Stationery Office, Edinburgh

Scottish Executive (May 2000) *The Same As You? A Review of Services for People with Learning Disabilities*.The Stationery Office, Edinburgh

Scottish Executive (1999) *Aiming for Excellence*.The Stationery Office, Edinburgh

Scottish Executive (1998) *Acute Services Review*.The Stationery Office, Edinburgh

Walker C, Ryan T, Walker A (1993). *Quality of Life after Resettlement for People with Learning Disabilities. Report to the North West Regional Health Authority,. Sheffield.* Department of Sociological Studies, University of Sheffield, Sheffield

Whoriskey M (1998) Quality of Life and Deinstitutionaliation—an evaluation of the effects of moving people with learning disabilities from hospital to live in the community. University of St Andrews

Wolfensberger W (1972). *The Principle of Normalisation in Human Services*. National Institute on Mental Retardation, Toronto

Wolfensberger W, Glenn L (1975) *PASS 3: A Method for the Quantitative Education of Human Services*. National Institute of Mental Retardation,Toronto

Wolfensberger W, Thomas S (1983) *PASSING: Program Analysis of Service Systems Implementation of Normalisation Goals*. National Institute of Mental Retardation, Toronto

5
Genetics and ethics: The way forward

Walter Muir

Introduction

Genetics and ethics are both seemingly complex areas when applied to the conditions associated with learning disability, and it is easy to interpret aspects of each as being mutually exclusive. Integration must come between them, but will take time, especially when the pace of change in the former seems to outstrip the development of the latter. It is widely agreed that ethical guidelines and principals, on how we obtain and use the knowledge and discoveries arising out of recent developments in molecular genetics, must not be developed solely by geneticists or scientists alone, but should involve participation from all levels in society, including people with learning disability themselves and those who care for them. However, such participation is made difficult both by the rate of change and the language and symbolism surrounding it. It is hoped, in the brief space allotted, to give some understanding of genetics and its recent developments, how these relate to learning disability, and to discuss some of the ethical issues that arise.

Learning disability

Learning disability is the term we now use in the UK to describe a collection of cognitive developmental outcomes that arise from a multitude of causes. As we usually interpret the term, it suggests that the person has some significant impairment of his or her cognitive abilities (or, less helpfully, 'intelligence'—with an IQ of 70 or less being significantly different from the population average) that becomes apparent during childhood, and out of which has emerged a significant degree of difficulty with social adaptation, usually manifest by problems with a variety of aspects of day-to-day living. This definition is widely accepted throughout the world, and more and more commonly given its proper place as a qualifying statement.

The terms 'disability' and 'handicap' are often confused as being synonymous. In the World Health Organization's definition, handicap is reserved for the personal or social disadvantage that may or may not result from a disability (... a restriction or lack of an ability to perform an activity in the manner, or within the range considered to be normal). The disability itself results from impairment. Here we have a series of causes and outcomes that may or may not be made apparent. Whether the impairment is such to lead to disability and the disability to handicap depends on the severity of the impairment, the intrinsic adaptive and compensatory mechanisms available to the person and also, crucially, on his or her personal, cultural and social environment. It is only in this full context that disability can become handicap, and the handicap understood.

Learning disability is not then a primary disorder; it is a descriptor of certain (very important) features that are secondary to a range of underlying developmental disturbances, which can be the consequence of an enormous variety of underlying developmental impairments. In the United States, for instance, the main and very widely used medical diagnostic manual (DSM-IV-TR) has no disorder that represents learning disability, but instead defines this on a secondary qualifier axis (they in fact use the term 'mental retardation' and 'learning disability' has a completely different meaning in this context, which has been a source of considerable confusion). However, to say that a person *has* a learning disability, in the sense that this is primary, has often been implied, in large part due to the lack of knowledge of the relevant condition(s) leading to the intellectual, social and developmental triage that define the name. The point is worth labouring as the misreading of learning disability (or any of the previous terminology) as a disorder in itself has been, in the past, one part of the mislabelling and maltreatment of whole sections of society, and continuing usage of the term 'learning disability' as having primary explanatory power does the person an injustice. Unfortunately, this type of reasoning is still present in some areas, such as our definition of mental impairment being 'a disorder' in the various current UK mental health legislatures. The more general use of the term in this sense denies important inter- and intra-individual variability and uniqueness.

In the past, it has restricted the search for prognostic outcomes that are useful to the person, based on the individual's reaction to the presence of specific, proximate, underlying disorders. We increasingly need to find, characterise and understand these underlying conditions so that we can best maximise all the potentials of the individual who has them. It is quite clear that many of these conditions will have a genetic basis and that we are poised, through the dramatic recent acceleration in the development of tools to study our molecular underpinnings, at the edge of a knowledge explosion about how genes influence all aspects of our lives. Such knowledge will certainly throw up new ethical challenges and raise the spectre of old abuses. It is up to us to make sure we understand the genetic concepts involved, so that we can play an informed part in making decisions as to the way ahead. There are two possible dangers here; firstly, that we make ethical policy decisions where we misunderstand the genetic arguments; and, secondly, where advances in ethics are unable to keep pace with advances in genetics. Genetic concepts are not difficult to understand; that they appear to be so is due to the shorthand and jargon, essential to rapid information exchange within any scientific discipline. Understanding the concepts is important to non-geneticists and this chapter, in the very brief space allowed, will attempt to explain some of those relevant to people with learning disability.

The importance of understanding proximate causes that lead to the outcome of learning disability

In recent decades, something of a change has taken place in the nature of the underlying conditions that have learning disability as one outcome. The number of people for whom learning disability is an outcome of infection or trauma has decreased (at least in developed countries) and the proportion of genetic conditions that contribute to the whole has increased. This is not to say that non-genetic causes are no longer important—severe prematurity and the foetal alcohol syndrome are just two such causes that are being increasingly recognised, but there are no longer the great numbers of infantile or childhood meningo-encephalitis, and there is little doubt that genetic factors play a major role in determining the cognitive outcome for many.

The clearest case, at present, where knowledge of the underlying condition does make a difference is where learning disability arises in people with Down's syndrome. Knowing that a person has Down's syndrome allows us to make predictions in comparison to people without Down's syndrome; individuals are at higher risk of congenital heart or bowel conditions, thyroid disorders are especially common, there is a much greater chance of developing a dementia when still relatively young, and these are but a few. Knowing the altered risks increases our awareness of these problems in the person, allows us to plan for their early detection and implementation of strategies to try and minimise their impact on the person's life. Knowing the proximate causes of the learning disability, however, also has other consequences. It is one part of the jigsaw to be fitted together when we are trying to find out why a person does not develop these outcomes, while the underlying cause is still definitely present—the buffers that the person has, against the stresses with which the condition loads the person.

Let's stay with the example posed by people with Down's syndrome. This is (at present) the most common genetic, non-inherited condition associated with learning disability. In most cases, it is due to the presence of three rather than the usual two copies of chromosome 21 in the person's cells (thus trisomy 21). In most people with Down's syndrome, every single nucleated cell in the person's body will have three copies of this chromosome. However, not every person will have all the associates of Down's syndrome and great differences will be found. These differences are determined by the interplay between the differential genetics (remember there are still twenty two other pairs of chromosomes in addition to chromosome 21) and other factors in the internal environment, the person's upbringing, experiences and interactions during development, and the social and cultural inheritance and environment in which the person is immersed. In the past, a failure to realise that there is no such thing as absolute genetic determinism has been the source of much genetic pseudo-science. We need to try and understand all these facets to be able to go beyond statistical predictions of risk, and to devise targeted interventions to negate the risks for the person with Down's syndrome—and understanding the genetic underpinnings that they contribute is equally important in this process, as it is in the other areas. This holistic approach goes beyond ascribing primacy to one area or another—something that has been quite prevalent—and engendered much conflict in those who support the extreme medical or social models of learning disability, where either the biological or the social are sufficient in themselves to explain the totality of the situation. In saying this, it is interesting to note that the number of genes in trisomy on chromosome 21, which play an important role in determining the various clinical features of Down's syndrome, may be much less than the entire gene complement of chromosome 21, and actually open to analysis (Epstein, 2002); thus, laying a foundation for finding ways to reduce the risk of common outcomes, such as thyroid disorder, perhaps even dementia, even if we still have a long way to go to fathom the complexities involved in the generation of the associated learning disability.

However, genetics does open up other areas of investigation that are less clearly beneficial in many cases, and the issues have a much wider impact than simply for learning disability.

This is especially so for genetic testing. At this point it is perhaps wise to summarise some of the concepts of genetics.

A brief genetic primer

Originally, genetics referred to the study of inheritance and those aspects of the person or organism determined in the main part by heredity, that is, passed on from one's parents. More recently, its meaning has been widened and now includes in its widest scale, evolutionary genetics and population genetics, through to molecular genetics of specific organisms (especially in mouse, fruit fly, zebra fish, worm—where genetic manipulation is relatively easy or its results easy to follow— through to biology), and the clinically relevant molecular genetics of body systems (neurogenetics, ophthalmic genetics, etc), diseases (cancer genetics, genetic endocrinology, etc), and therapeutic strategies (pharmacogenetics (Roses, 2000)). The range is bewildering and permeates all aspects of medicine. In fact, since no disease is without genetic underpinnings at some level, the textbook of medicine of the future is likely to be based on molecular principles (Beaudet *et al*, 2001).

In humans, the basic units of inheritance are genes found within the cell nucleus, and determine the sequence of amino acids that are joined to create proteins in the cell. Genes are functional units within the great linear stretches of a linked molecular necklace, where the individual beads take one of four forms of chemicals termed nucleotides (the whole is termed deoxyribosenucleic acid or more commonly DNA). This, with associated structural proteins, is the basis of twenty-three discrete chromosome pairs (the 'diploid count') present in all our nucleated cells, with the exception of germ cells (gametes; ova and sperm), which have only half this number ('haploid count'), to be made diploid again when fused with a gamete from the opposite sex at conception. The flow of information is from gene to protein via a complementary necklace made from a slightly different chemical (ribosenucleic acid or RNA). RNA intermediates transfer the information from the cell's nucleus to the protein-assembly factories in the cytoplasm (ribosomes). Both genes, and the RNA intermediates they make, can be subject to disruptions that lead to disease. For simplicity, we will restrict discussion to disruptions of the gene.

One of the twenty-three chromosome pairs is special—the sex chromosomes are dimorphic in type, women having two X chromosomes, men having an X chromosome and a Y chromosome. When most cells divide, the chromosome number is doubled then shared evenly between the two daughter cells (mitotic division) so as to maintain the correct gene complement. In the germ cells (ova and sperm), however, there is no doubling and each individual cell contains half the number of chromosomes (meiotic division), a situation that means that the full complement is restored on fertilisation of the ovum by a sperm. Meiosis also differs in that the chromosomes (each pair with their corresponding partner and stretches of DNA) are exchanged between the pair. This process—recombination—is essential to maintain a trans-generational level of variation in the DNA segregating from the parents to the child. The further apart two pieces of DNA lie on a chromosome, the less likely they are to recombine—a fact that is made use of in various forms of genetic analysis. Genes from one parent may be partnered with genes from the other in a huge number of different ways. Each individual gene may show different expression levels or other characteristics due to its innate genetic sequence variability (allelic variation), which also results from recombination through generations. This variation is, in fact, highly important to species survival; it means that, within a population, there is enough gene variability to permit adaptation to changing environmental conditions. That some variations may seem 'harmful' is only true within a given set of environmental circumstances and time frames. The main point is that recombination (and its necessary outcome-random gene assortment) and other changes directed at the genes DNA sequence (*mutations*) are natural phenomena essential to the long-term survival of any species. Of course, structural changes in genes can occur in unnatural ways—through the influence of radiation, teratogenic drugs (that are harmful to an embryo), etc—and these are, in the bulk of cases, harmful and unwanted. However, it is likely that many changes in DNA sequence do not give rise to harmful or even apparent outcomes. Whether they do or do not, they may be passed on from one generation to the next and, in doing so, the observable outcome within a family depends on the fact that we normally have two chromosomes of each type and, thus, two active copies of the same type of gene. When disruption of only one copy of the gene is needed to produce an effect, this indicates that the amount of protein produced from the other active gene is insufficient to compensate (a situation called haploinsufficiency). Only one copy of the inactive gene then needs be inherited for a condition to be expressed and the inheritance is said to be *dominant*. Every generation of a family is likely to have affected members. If the genes on each of the chromosomes of a given pair have to be affected before a condition is seen, then the inheritance is said to follow a *recessive* pattern. It requires inheritance of gene mutations from *each* parent and, either the rate of new gene mutation in a population must be high for more common recessive conditions, or there may be a familial relationship between the parents when the gene mutation is very rare (thus, some recessive conditions are more common in groups where cousin marriages are more common). Since the parents are unaffected, the smaller size of nuclear families in Western countries has meant that many recessive conditions appear as if 'out of the blue'. The dominant and recessive forms of inheritance were originally described by Mendel, and are termed classical Mendelian types.

However, it is more often the case that the clinical outcome of a disrupted gene does not fit neatly into one of these classes—*partial dominance*—where other factors (genetic and non-genetic) that modify the clinical picture are far more common. Genes on the sex chromosomes prove exceptions to this picture. The Y chromosome is largely devoid of genes, so most mutations for genes on the X chromosome in males have a clinical outcome. This phenomenon plays a large part in the excess of men who have a learning disability. In women, one or other X chromosome is inactivated in a random fashion, so that some cells will express a fully normal gene; in others, the mutated gene will be on the activated chromosome, and so the clinical picture for women tends to be much less severe. Inheritance of mutations of genes on the X chromosome, thus, tends to follow a distinctive pattern, with affected males much more common than females, and with no transmission from fathers to sons (they can only pass on their Y chromosome).

The human genetic material has been sequenced in draft (Lander *et al*, 2001; Venter *et al*, 2001) and the detailed annotation and description in full of each chromosome is coming on stream. We already know how many genes there are in an entire human genome—around 40 000. This is much fewer than initially thought, but the RNAs and the proteins they code for are often spliced together in different ways to greatly increase the repertoire of different types. Mutations in DNA may affect splicing of RNA; thus, protein formation and a recent class of disorders has been created on the basis of these, including nervous system disorders, such as forms of frontotemporal dementia with parkinsonism (Cartegni *et al*, 2002). A large percentage of these genes are expressed (the term used for when genes are 'switched on' to make proteins) in the brain and, thus, involved in its development and activity (Cravchik *et al*, 2001). The function of many is still unknown and their biological role remains to be clarified.

Disrupting the DNA sequence—gene mutations, through to chromosomal abnormalities

Strictly, a mutation is defined as any change in the linear sequence of nucleotides in DNA. If such a change alters the sequence within in a gene, then it may alter the structure of the protein that the gene codes for, which may, in turn, alter the individual's functioning. Mutations can occur at a wide variety of levels. Originally, they were held to be of stable inheritance and unchanging from one generation to the next. Many of the earlier genetic discoveries were of rare, simple mutations in genes for important enzymes (the 'inborn errors of metabolism'). A substitution of one base for another in the sequence of DNA in a gene may change the amino acid that the particular part of the gene codes for—the protein structure changes and this may impair function. However, we now know that some mutations—dynamic mutations—are unstable in size across generations. The key example here is from the Fragile X syndrome. This fairly common X-linked condition affects around 1 in 4000 men and half as many women.

Many mutations have no effect on the gene's ability to code for a protein (null mutations), but others cause an abnormal protein to be generated (mis-sense mutations). Mutations can range from changes in the type of nucleotide present at a single point in the DNA chain (a single base pair mutation), through deletions of large stretches of a chromosome involving many genes, to an entire absence or duplication of a chromosome where the expression of large numbers of genes is altered. The number of genes that are involved in nervous system development and function is a very large percentage of the total number of human genes. Thus, the nervous system is very likely to be affected when a gene is disrupted in some way. It should be no surprise, then, that the number of genetic conditions affecting the nervous system, and also producing a learning disability, is huge. By grouping these conditions on the basis of an (exceptionally important) cognitive outcome, we are linking together a countless variety of different conditions that, in other ways, can be very dissimilar.

Most chromosomal abnormalities that have clinical effect can be thought of as large-scale mutations involving the duplication or deletion of large numbers of genes at once (some translocations, however, may only disrupt a single gene at a breakpoint).

A very large number of different chromosome re-arrangements and numerical abnormalities have been described (many are very rare) and many are not associated with learning disability (Keitges and Luthardt, 2001). More recently, smaller re-arrangements that are on the verge of, or escape, the resolution of normal microscopy have been defined and form an important group of conditions that lead to learning disability (Shaffer *et al*, 2001). These tend to disrupt several genes at once. Prader-Willi syndrome is an example that occurs on chromosome 15, where learning disability of a variable degree is associated with a hyperphagia—an increase in appetite (Cassidy *et al*, 2000), Williams syndrome on chromosome 7—with its distinctive cognitive profile (Harris, 1998), and the Velocardiofacial syndrome on chromosome 22, which is thought to be associated with both learning disability and schizophrenia (Scambler, 2000). DNA that is complementary to the region of interest can be labelled with a fluorophore and hybridised to the chromosome in question (FISH—fluorescence *in situ* hybridisation). Under the fluorescent microscope, deletions can be seen by a lack of fluorescence and changes well below the level of light microscopy seen. A whole series of re-arrangements near the ends of chromosomes (telomeres) has been described in a percentage of children with previously unexplained learning disability (Knight *et al*, 1999).

Returning to Down's syndrome, it also illustrates issues around pre-natal testing for a genetic disorder. The test itself need not be based on DNA and, for Downs syndrome, it has for many years centred on an altered level of a maternal blood component—alpha foeto protein (and, more recently, two other proteins—human chorionic gonadotropin and beta oestradiol), which is associated with an increased risk (not absolute) of carrying a foetus with trisomy 21. Testing is coupled to the significantly increased risk of trisomy where maternal age is over 35 years, an association that has been long known, where it is becoming more clear that the error usually occurs during maternal meiosis and may be associated with abnormal chiasma formation, but the full reason is still unknown. Further checks involve histopathology—the analysis of foetal cells obtained directly by chorionic villus sampling or from the amniotic fluid (amniocentesis). None of this, note, involves examining DNA from the foetus or the mother directly. The outcome of such tests is still at present to allow the parents to make a choice about whether to continue with the pregnancy.

Similarly, for newborns, one of most important and earliest tests for a genetic disorder associated with learning disability was (is) one of the oldest tests—Guthries inhibition assay for the presence of phenylketonuria (PKU). Again, this test predated the present era of DNA testing and has resulted in a dramatic change in the quality of life expected for people who have PKU, inasmuch as avoidance of phenylalanine in the diet means that the harmful effects of the condition on brain development and, thus learning disability, are largely avoided. The case of PKU signals a precautionary note for all tests, prenatal or newborn. Before its biology was known, PKU could lead to disastrous consequences for the person, including blindness, profound learning disability and epilepsy. Knowing the biology led to treatment (in this case dietary avoidance) and showed that treatment after birth is not too late in this case to prevent severe learning disability. PKU is caused by mutations in a single gene; many conditions associated with learning disability are much more complex, but, as we unravel their biology, means of countering the unwanted and deleterious effects of the gene mutations are likely to be found (Lindee, 2000).

At present, most prenatal testing is done in the context of allowing parents to choose whether to continue pregnancy rather than for predicting treatment needs and necessary interventions to maximise the quality of life for the individual, and it is sometimes forgotten in arguments against prenatal testing that the knowledge required to create such tests may also play an important part in developing treatment rationales. Discrimination against people with learning disability is not a necessary or inevitable outcome of prenatal diagnosis, or rather its assumed consequence of termination, but it does certainly have the potential to produce significant negative outcomes; and it must be accepted that many groups, including those with learning disability may find it distressing or offensive (Gillam, 1999). One valid problem area lies in the, often, extensive delays (in some cases perhaps interminable) between our ability to detect and ability to treat. The so called 'new genetics' amplifies both aspects discussed here, detection and understanding of biology, rather than fundamentally change the situation. At present, however, it is fair to say that, in the coming few years, disorder detection will greatly outpace our fundamental understandings of the chain of events that lead from gene abnormalities to a cognitive syndrome, such as learning disability.

Advances in technology

Advances in biotechnology have driven many of the recent advances in genetics. The polymerase chain reaction (PCR) allows the specific amplification of short stretches of DNA from tiny amounts of sample. If the short, specific, amplified stretches contain a gene or part of a gene, then a simple method can be designed to amplify (and at the same time isolate it) so that it can be readily examined to see if it contains a sequence error—*a mutation*. PCR amplification, along with methodologies of mutation detection, form the basis of most DNA-based 'genetic tests' for genetic disorders associated with learning disability. 'Cloning' is the term used for the insertion of pieces of DNA of one species into another biological agent (usually into the DNA of a microorganism, such as a bacterium or a simple organism, such as yeast—the host for the extraneous DNA is usually called a vector) that can then be manipulated in various ways to study the particular stretch of DNA in question. The combination of the two methods is very powerful. Cloning and sequencing have led to the isolation of large numbers of DNA sequence polymorphisms that vary between unrelated individuals, but are of stable inheritance within families. These form the basis for modern methods of finding the chromosomal locus for the suspected disease genes that are inherited in families. Recently, there has been a focus on polymorphisms that involve only one nucleotide in a sequence rather than a run of such bases. These single nucleotide polymorphisms (SNPs) are widely distributed throughout the genome, easily identified in a DNA sample (a process called typing), and very large numbers are now detailed in public (and commercial) databases (Nowotny *et al*, 2001) The chromosomal position of such polymorphisms can be identified in the various family members, then tests applied to see if it significantly associates with the disorder down generations. If it does, then it is likely to lie near the gene for the disorder, since we have already noted that recombination between chromatids increases with separation between two loci. The polymorphism is said to be linked to the gene and the methods, those of linkage analysis. The position of many inherited disorders has been identified by this method, and the easy manipulation of DNA by cloning has allowed rapid identification of the particular gene involved. Awareness of the structural changes in the given gene that lead to disorder means that rapid, specific PCR based assays for these mutations can be devised and analysed on very small samples. Usually, whole blood is used, since the nuclei of white cells are a rich source of DNA. A small venous blood sample can be used to generate DNA sufficient for many hundreds, perhaps thousands, of such assays using PCR based methods.

Techniques are being developed that allow the isolation of foetal cells that leak across the placenta into the maternal circulation. If this could be perfected, then a non-invasive (for the foetus at least), sensitive and specific means of testing for the presence of genetic disorders would emerge. Obviously, this would markedly increase the power of prenatal testing, and acutely magnify the possible ethical problems encountered when conditions, for which there is still no treatment available, are identified. Another important development has been the microarray, or, more colloquially, the 'DNA chip'. These employ microscale methods to form a grid of thousands of DNA types on a glass or other substrate, which can then be scanned rapidly for changes and differences. In this way, large scale detection of gene mutations is, in prospect, coupled to high throughput of samples using robotic methods. The possibilities for large population scale testing will obviously raise new ethical questions. Not only DNA can be micro-arrayed; there is an intensive effort to identify the presence of all proteins acting at a point in time in a given tissue using chip technology, which would lead to major advances in understanding complex biological system interactions (Service, 2001).

One strong candidate for chip technology would be to detect the X chromosome gene mutations associated with learning disability. For over a hundred years, it has been known that there is an excess of men with moderate to severe learning disability and that this is, in general, due to conditions linked to disturbed gene function on the X chromosome. There are few genes on the Y chromosome and, save for certain pseudoautosomal regions mutations on the X chromosomes, in men, usually lead to absence of gene product. In women, the sex chromosomes are unusual in that one of the pair of X chromosomes is near totally inactivated, but usually in a random fashion, so that around 50% of active chromosomes will contain the non-mutated gene (Avner and Heard, 2001). Therefore, women often show much less (or no) effect of an X linked condition compared to men; X linked conditions are thought to be the basis of the cause of the cognitive impairment in up to 20% of men with learning disability (Chelly and Mandel, 2001). Some of these are associated with other clinical features (the so called syndromic X linked mental retardations—MRXS), but a sizeable and increasing number have learning disability as the only detectable feature (MRX).

Again, the biology is now starting to emerge for some X-linked conditions and this is linking some conditions together. Rett syndrome, a learning disability associated X-linked condition largely expressed in women, is now known to be due to mutations in the gene MEPC2 (Zoghbi and Francke, 2001). Different mutations in the same gene have been found in a series of families with other MRX disorders, and the overall incidence of learning disability associated with MECP2 mutations may match that of Fragile X (Couvert *et al*, 2001).

Ethical issues and dilemmas

The major danger engendered by such genetic advances is based on the much wider perception (or misperception) that people with learning disability are, in some intrinsic way, physically and morally different from the rest of the population, a concept that leads to discrimination and the creation of an underclass. Byrne, in an exceptionally clear monograph, presents and rejects the arguments of recent philosophers who, by invoking such classificatory mechanisms, seek to reduce the worth of people with learning disability (Byrne, 2000). Byrne argues, deeply and convincingly, that people with a learning disability must have an equal moral status to all others through the fact of our common humanity, and deals with those who would argue that this is open to the charge of speciesism. More controversially for some, he also addresses the issue of termination and posits that policies of non-conception with respect to the prevention of the occurrence of cognitively disabled infants do not endorse genocidal policies or discriminatory attitudes towards existing disabled people. However, he also concedes that there may be no definitive answer to whether the early human foetus constitutes a human being with equal moral worth to all others. In fact, there may never be an accepted scientific answer to this question, with the concept always left to be defined by societal values and worth. The fact that some philosophers still exist who argue for a lower moral worth for people with learning disability is to some (including the present author) deeply disquieting.

Most assume that, originally, eugenics was a phenomenon restricted to Nazi Germany. This was not the case. The eugenic movement within the United States, for example, was well established in the early decades of the last century. The first eugenic sterilization law was passed in Indiana in 1907 and later 30 states passed similar legislation (Micklos and Carlson, 2000). The assumption that eugenic policies towards the learning disabled ceased after 1945 is also untrue. In Canada, Sweden and Switzerland, eugenic-based sterilization continued into the 1960s; in fact, as a post war politic, the ideas have shown a rather tenacious survival. In the UK, genetic counsellors have a careful rationale when advising parents on the genetic risks of having a child with a serious disability, which is to give the parents enough unbiased information to make their own decision—the principle of non-directiveness. Worryingly, Wertz has shown that non-directiveness may not be a norm that is held in all countries (Wertz, 2002). In a survey of 36 countries, she found that, save in North America, the UK and parts of Northern Europe, a practice of 'directive pessimism' was more often the presentation (Wertz, 1998). As the power of genetics makes detection of conditions that lead to learning disability simpler and more reliable, strict ethical safeguards will have to be in place to prevent such intentional or unintentional influences on parental decisions. Although not directly concerned with learning disability, the recent document 'Genetics and human behaviour: the ethical context', from the Nuffield Council on Bioethics covers these issues in an especially wide ranging and detailed way; it makes essential reading (Bioethics, 2002).

For people with learning disability, themselves, a number of other issues arise, and again these are not restricted to genetic concerns. Protection for the adult and child during investigations, treatment and research is based on the principles of mental capacity and autonomy, with autonomy preserved through the principle of informed consent. For some adults with learning disability, and for children, informed consent is not possible. This creates a well-recognised impasse between preservation of autonomy, and the need for treatments and understanding of the conditions involved, so as to find ways of maximising the person's potential. Various legislation has sought to come to terms with it. After the Second World War, the Code of Nurenberg, in 1947, forbade children and incapable adults from participation in research (Knoppers *et al*, 2002).

Although certainly understandable, this seriously curtailed the acquisition of knowledge relating to the conditions that result in a learning disability. Today, the view (but by no means a universal one) is tending towards recognition that such research is permissible, if it is minimally invasive and not directly harmful to the patient, and where research on a person without the specific condition leading to the learning disability would not give the required information. The Adults with Incapacity (Scotland) Act, 2000 makes this point, both allowing inclusion of individual while protecting their rights. At present, there is no such explicit system in England and Wales, and the situation in other countries is unclear.

Another possible source of discrimination, and one that worries many people, is that of differential insurance policies for those where the genetic makeup suggests a significant risk of developing a disorder. Since most genetic conditions run in families, the finding in one person has an influence beyond the individual sphere. Huntington's disease, for instance, is a dominantly inherited neuro-degenerative disorder with a late onset, and nearly all those carrying the mutated gene eventually showing the disorder. It is due to an alteration in a gene on the short arm of chromosome 4 that normally codes for the protein called huntingtin. Since, in its classical form, Huntington's disease is clinically apparent only when the subject is 40 to 50 years old, most carriers will have passed on the condition to a percentage of their children by the time it is detected. However, it can now be directly genetically tested for in persons of any age by examining the gene's DNA sequence. The testing has been possible for a decade now and has caused (and still does cause) numerous ethical dilemmas for the families concerned (Morris *et al*, 1989). At present, there is no cure for the condition and many do not wish to be made aware of their risk. They may also wish not to have others in the family made aware, if they carry the disorder. Under such circumstances, counselling and investigation needs to done on a family-by-family basis. However, there are more general guidelines; for instance, it is usually considered that if non-disclosure would mean putting other members of the family at risk of serious harm, then the principle of absolute confidentiality of medical information could and should be breached (Knoppers, 2002). This is different from refraining from forcing genetic information onto a person who does not him/herself wish to know and it is unlikely that valid exceptions exist to this principle (some might argue that this may be reasonable in cases involving reproductive risk rather than risk only to the given person). Again, these issues have direct relevance to genetic conditions that lead to learning disability in spite of the difference in the age at onset of the condition.

Issues also arise from the current potential to store DNA indefinitely (Deschenes *et al*, 2001). DNA is stable at low temperatures over many years and, since examining its structure requires ever diminishing sample sizes, then even a small amount can go a long way. In the clinical setting, DNA is usually obtained from the nuclei of a person's white blood cells and, by isolating such cells and treating them in vitro with a strain of the Epstein Barr Virus, the usual limits on the number of divisions a cell can make before it dies are removed and the cells are potentially immortalized. Although a fairly costly process, a self-replenishing store of cells can be created supplying DNA in relatively large amounts for extended periods of time. DNA can also be extracted from a wide variety of tissues other than human blood. Hair follicles, buccal cells from mouthwash samples, and skin cells are only a few in fairly common use. DNA can then easily outlive the person, and questions of tissue ownership arise. Some legal experts would prefer ethical guidelines rather than legislation on such issues (Skene, 2002); others argue towards the continued complete personal ownership of any separated part of the body.

The easy availability of DNA combines with the ease of mutation detection to mean that simple DNA tests for a rapidly expanding number of conditions are feasible. The most difficult situation is where these tests are predictive of disorders for which there are no current treatments, raising the possibility of insurance discrimination against those who will develop substantial health and social care needs. Even with recent advances for most conditions that produce a learning disability, there is no treatment that reverses this outcome. The best insurance against discrimination in this respect is a national policy on health and social input to meet the needs of the most disadvantaged, but this is far from universal. At present in the UK, there is a moratorium on the use of most genetic tests in insurance estimations. However, this is unlikely to continue. Affiliated to genetic testing for disorders is genetic pharmaco-profiling, where the person's intrinsic genetic background is used to define the best genetically matched therapies (most effective, least side effects) for a given disorder. This need not be a genetic condition in itself. An antibiotic for an infection could, for instance, be selected on the basis of a person's rate of metabolising a given drug, which is often highly genetically determined (Roses, 2000). This, like all the other developments in genetics, raises contentious issues. The use of specialized treatments for only small groups might in itself produce new stigmatising clusters; in addition, it might fragment the therapeutic market, leading to more expensive treatments designed for fewer and fewer people (Rothstein and Epps, 2001).

Although genetics is increasing in diagnostic power, we may over interpret its overall importance. Steve Jones, a distinguished geneticist, has pointed out:

> *'It has been said that the four letters of the genetic code are H, Y, P and E and medical providers must realize that the molecular biology business is as adept at promoting its wares as is any other".*
>
> (Jones, 2000)

It has been noted already that scientists alone should not be making the ethical policy decisions with regards to genetic advances. In fact, the general public's perceptions will be important in deciding the way ahead. It is, therefore, useful to try and understand what the public perceive to be the ethical issues involved. Kerr and her colleagues have addressed such issues and some of the public perceptions make sobering reading (Kerr *et al*, 1998a; 1998b). Far from being without views or lacking in expertise about genetics, they often have very strong opinions (not necessarily based on scientific fact), with a significant level of scepticism and ambivalence about both professional (medical doctors in this case) and governmental accountability. In particular, they found that the groups they investigated thought treatments for genetic conditions to be more palatable than termination, but perceived a current lack of care for people with genetic disorders, and that the boundaries between good and bad practice were often unclear. The tendency to imply that the public do not ('need more public education') or cannot understand the issues, bypasses them in the decision making process. It is something that cannot be justified and incorporating, as well as improving, the lay understanding of genetics of learning disability is vital to ethical progress.

References

Avner P, Heard E (2001) X-chromosome inactivation: counting, choice and initiation. *Nat Rev Genet* **2**: 59–67.

Beaudet AL, Scriver CR, Sly WS, Valle D (2001) Genetics, biochemistry, and molecular bases of variant human phenotypes. In: Scriver CR, Beaudet AL, Sly WS *et al*, eds. *The Metabolic and Molecular Bases of Inherited Disease*. McGraw-Hill, New York: 3–45

Bioethics, Nuffield Council on (2002) *Genetics and Human Behaviour: The Ethical Context*. Nuffield Council on Bioethics, London: 220

Byrne PJ (2000) *Philosophical and Ethical Problems in Mental Handicap*. Macmillan Press, Basingstoke

Cartegni L, Chew SL, Krainer AR (2002) Listening to silence and understanding nonsense: exonic mutations that affect splicing. *Nat Rev Genet* **3**: 285–98

Cassidy SB, Dykens E, Williams CA (2000) Prader-Willi and Angelman syndromes: sister imprinted disorders. *Am J Med Genet* **97**: 136–46

Chelly J, Mandel JL (2001) Monogenic causes of X-linked mental retardation. *Nat Rev Genet* **2**: 669–80

Couvert P, Bienvenu T, Aquaviva C *et al* (2001) MECP2 is highly mutated in X-linked mental retardation. *Hum Mol Genet* **10**: 941–46

Cravchik A, Subramanian G, Broder S, Venter JC (2001) Sequence analysis of the human genome: implications for the understanding of nervous system function and disease. *Arch Neurol* **58**: 1772–78

Deschenes M, Cardinal G, Knoppers BM, Glass KC (2001) Human genetic research, DNA banking and consent: a question of 'form'? *Clin Genet* **59**: 221–39

Epstein CJ (2002. From Down syndrome to the 'Human' in 'Human Genetics'. *Am J Hum Genet* **70**: 300–13

Gillam L (1999) Prenatal diagnosis and discrimination against the disabled. *J Med Ethics* **25**: 163–71

Harris JC (1998) Williams (Williams-Beuren) Syndrome. In: *Developmental Neuropsychiatry*. Oxford University Press, New York: 319–32

Jones S (2000) *Genetics in Medicine: Real Promises, Unreal Expectations. One Scientist's Advice to Policymakers in the United Kingdom and the United States*. Milbank Memorial Fund, New York

Keitges E, Luthardt FW (2001) Human Chromosomes. In: *Encyclopedia of Life Sciences*. Nature Publishing Group: 1–8; www.els.net

Kerr A, Cunningham-Burley S, Amos A (1998a) Drawing the line: an analysis of lay people's discussions about the new genetics. *Pub Underst Sci* **7**: 113–33

Kerr A, Cunningham-Burley S, Amos A (1998b) The new genetics and health: mobilizing lay expertise. *Pub Underst Sci* **7**: 41–60

Knight SJ, Regan R, Nicod A *et al* (1999) Subtle chromosomal rearrangements in children with unexplained mental retardation. *Lancet* **354**: 1676–81

Knoppers BM (2002) Genetic information and the family: are we our brother's keeper? *Trends Biotechnol* **20**: 85–86

Knoppers BM, Avard D, Cardinal G, Glass KC (2002). Science and society: children and incompetent adults in genetic research: consent and safeguards. *Nat Rev Genet* **3**: 221–25

Lander ES, Linton LM, Birren B *et al* (2001) Initial sequencing and analysis of the human genome. *Nature* **409**: 860–921

Lindee MS (2000) Genetic disease since 1945. *Nat Rev Genet* **1**: 236–41

Micklos D, Carlson E (2000) Engineering American society: the lesson of eugenics. *Nat Rev Genet* **1**: 153–58

Morris MJ, Tyler A, Lazarou L, Meredith L, Harper PS (1989) Problems in genetic prediction for Huntington's disease. *Lancet* **2**: 601–603

Nowotny P, Kwon JM, Goate AM (2001) SNP analysis to dissect human traits. *Curr Opin Neurobiol* **11**: 637–41

Roses AD (2000). Pharmacogenetics and the practice of medicine. *Nature* **405**: 857–65

Rothstein MA, Epps PG (2001). Ethical and legal implications of pharmacogenomics. *Nat Rev Genet* **2**: 228–31

Scambler PJ (2000) The 22q11 deletion syndromes. *Hum Mol Genet* **9**: 2421–26

Service RF (2001) Proteomics. Searching for recipes for protein chips. *Science* **294**: 2080–82

Shaffer LG, Ledbetter DH, Lupski JR (2001) Molecular cytogenetics of contiguous gene syndromes: mechanisms and consequences of gene dosage imbalance. In: Scriver CR, Beaudet AL, Sly WS, *et al*, eds. *The Metabolic & Molecular Bases of Inherited Disease*. McGraw-Hill, New York: 1291–324

Skene L (2002) Ownership of human tissue and the law. *Nat Rev Genet* **3**: 145–48

Venter JC, Adams MD, Myers EW, *et al* (2001) The sequence of the human genome. *Science* **291**: 1304–51

Wertz DC (2002) Ethics watch: Did eugenics ever die? *Nat Rev Genet* **3**: 408

Wertz DC (1998) Eugenics is alive and well: a survey of genetic professionals around the world. *Sci Context* **11**: 493–510

Zoghbi HY, Francke U (2001) Rett Syndrome. In: Scriver CR, Beaudet AL, Sly WS, *et al*, eds. *The Metabolic & Molecular Bases of Inherited Disease*. McGraw-Hill, New York: 6329–38

6

Integration: The legal issues; *past, present and future*

Ros Lyall

This chapter will consider the important legal issues that impact on the lives of people with learning disabilities and give a broad overview of the legislative and regulatory framework within which both those providing and receiving health care have to function. The scale of legislative change in the recent past, which has impacted in some way or other on the lives of people with learning disabilities, is considerable. The principles by which governments and society set legislation are similar throughout the Western world, although there are some glaring anomalies. It is only very recently that the US courts have acknowledged that it is unlawful to execute 'mentally retarded criminals'. Within the United Kingdom, we are required to work with legislation enacted by the European Union, as well as with Westminster and devolved powers in Scotland, Wales and Northern Ireland.

It is also important to note that this is an ever-changing picture and much of what could be written is likely to be out of date within a very short space of time, the detail superseded by newer legislation. This is particularly relevant to any discussion on Mental Health legislation where, in both Scotland, England and Wales, there are current parliamentary and national debates about proposed new mental health acts.

History

The history of legislation in respect of people with a learning disability has largely mirrored the view that society, as a whole, has at any given time. Until the late 1880s, legislation affecting people with a learning disability was largely concerned with the management of their property. As early as King Edward I, the distinction had been made between those affected intermittently by incapacity and those who were incapable from birth. The rationale for this administrative split was in terms of property management. In the former case, the Crown managed the property only when the person was *non compos mentis*; in the latter, the estates, etc, fell to the crown for all time. There is little further major legislation in the UK until the nineteenth century. Then, in 1886, what is colloquially known as 'The Idiots Act' laid down regulations concerning the admission and discharge of people to institutional care, and also the registration and inspection of such establishments. As such, it marked the first piece of legislation to deal with the health and welfare of people with a learning disability and not just their property. It was enacted 40 years after the appearance of the first establishment in Britain based on the Abendberg, an institution founded to provide, for the first time, segregated (from those with mental illness) care for children with learning disabilities. It was founded on the belief that education and treatment would maximise the development of children with learning disabilities and it became the model for care across Europe and North America. Ironic then that the institutions spawned by the Abendberg, and indeed the Abendberg itself, were subject to allegations of cruelty and neglect throughout their existence. The Abendberg had been founded in the belief that education would lead to 'cure' and attainment of normality. When this inevitably proved an impossible goal, society's view of people with learning disability changed and the institutions, founded with such high ideals, became regarded as the depositories for undesirable elements of society.

The concerns of society about the quality of care and treatment led to the Idiots Act and have been the driving force behind many of the policy and legislative changes over the years. The pace of legislative change has quickened in the latter part of the twentieth century and early years of the twenty-first. The reasons for this can be found in the changing view of society with regard to many aspects of the human condition. Foremost among these are beliefs about human rights, abuse, power over one's own body, equality among peoples, rights to self expression etc, against a background, within learning disability circles, of normalisation, the wholesale closure of institutions, the right to be seen as a valued member of society, and the right to self determination. In the years following the Idiots Act, there were mental health acts in 1913 that remained in force until 1959/1960, and then a further reform in 1983/1984. As noted above, yet more reform is planned for 2003. Much of the legislation has been viewed as positive in its effect on the lives of people with a disability; some of it has promised much and delivered little, other aspects are now regarded as outdated, as thinking and aspiration moves on. Legislation governs rights to education, services, assessment (but not necessarily of provision to meet identified need), the right to vote, entitlement to benefit, rebates of statutory charges, such as the council tax, disability discrimination, and much more.

Within Scotland, there has been new legislation governing aspects of people's lives that have previously been subject to ad hoc and often inappropriate or legally invalid arrangements. The recent Adults with Incapacity Act (2000) is regarded by many as a genuine attempt to regularise various aspects of care, including the thorny question of consent to treatment for people who are incapable of making their own decisions. The legislation, which will be discussed in greater detail at a later point, includes people who are incapable because of age, mental illness, and physical disability resulting in an inability to communicate, as well as those with a learning disability who may be regarded as incapable. Not all adults with a learning disability will be covered by this legislation, as it seeks to maximise the extent to which people can retain control and autonomy.

Principles

The principals governing the majority of legislation are contained within broad statements issued by the World Health Organization, the United Nations, and the European Union, including the Court of Human Rights. These were codified in a resolution adopted by the United Nations General Assembly in 1971.

The Rights of the Mentally Retarded Person (sic) (abridged)
Adopted by the United Nations General Assembly 1971

- The same basic rights as other citizens of the same country and the same age
- The right to proper medical care ...education, training, habilitation and guidance as will enable him to develop his ability and potential to the fullest possible extent
- The right to economic security, a decent standard of living. The right to productive work or other meaningful occupation
- The right to live with his own family or with foster parents: to participate in all aspects of community life, be provided with appropriate leisure activities. If care in an institution becomes necessary, it should be in surroundings and under circumstances as close to normal living as possible
- The right to a qualified guardian when this is required to protect him
- The right to protection from exploitation, abuse and degrading treatment. If accused, the right to a fair trial with full recognition being given to his degree of responsibility
- Some may be unable, because of the severity of their handicap, to exercise for themselves all of their rights in a meaningful way. For others, modification of some or all of these rights is appropriate. The procedures used for the modification or denial of rights must contain proper legal safeguards against every form of abuse, must be based on an evaluation of the social capability of the person by qualified experts and must be subject to periodic reviews and the right of appeal to higher authorities
- Above all THE RIGHT TO RESPECT.

Mental health legislation

At the time of writing, mental health legislation in the United Kingdom is under review and new mental health bills for England and Wales, Scotland, but not Northern Ireland, are making their way through the respective parliamentary processes. Nevertheless, the principles contained within the legislation are broadly similar.

Despite vigorous campaigning by self-advocacy and voluntary organisations concerned with people with learning disabilities, the concept of a learning disability as a 'mental disorder' remains within the scope of the proposed legislation. There are powers to detain people in hospital and to treat against their will, albeit with considerable safeguards. The role of the Mental Welfare Commission in Scotland remains and with it a new proposal for Mental Health Tribunals. There is also a much stronger statement about 'reciprocity'. This is the principle whereby detained patients, at least have a right to expect that they will be provided with all appropriate care and treatment in reasonable surroundings. The actual delivery of this principle, which seems so straight forward, has major resource implications for the NHS in Scotland. In England and Wales, the proposals would appear to be rather more far-reaching and there has been considerable disquiet among professionals about the implications. Given the current uncertainty about mental health legislation in the United Kingdom, I propose to concentrate on consent to treatment issues as these also have a bearing on the Adults with Incapacity (Scotland) Act 2000.

Under current and proposed legislation, treatment for mental disorder is subject to a number of controls under existing mental health legislation. Generally, if you are an informal patient and consent to treatment, then the treatment will be given. The only circumstances where there is a requirement for additional consents from external bodies/professionals is in relation to treatment using psychosurgery or the implantation of sex hormones with the aim of reducing sex drive; in Scotland, this proviso only applies to detained patients. However, if you are a detained patient, then there are additional safeguards to ensure that you are not treated against your will. If you consent to a treatment contained within the regulations (treatment with psychotropic medication for more than three months, or ECT for example), then the doctor has to certify that you have so consented and notify the Mental Welfare Commission/Mental Health Act Commission appropriately. If you do not consent and the doctor still wishes to give you certain treatments, then they have to ask for a second opinion from a psychiatrist appointed by the Mental Welfare Commission/Mental Health Act Commission. These arrangements only cover treatment for mental disorder and not treatment for any physical illness. It does not appear as though these provisions are going to change dramatically in any new legislation.

Consent to treatment for other medical treatment is now subject to very different rules in the constituent parts of the UK. Legislation pertaining to this has been enacted in Scotland as discussed below, but in England and Wales there is no equivalent legal framework.

The Adults with Incapacity (Scotland) Act 2000

I make no apology for concentrating on a major piece of legislation from a small country in the northern half of Europe that has only recently achieved some devolution of power and authority from central government control. One of the major achievements of devolution has been the increased ability of Scotland to determine its own legislative framework. It always did have its own legal system, but all too often, legislation created for England and Wales was merely 'tartanised, and no account taken of the differences north of the border.

In Scotland, the move to close large institutions for people with a learning disability has lagged behind England and Wales. Nevertheless, there is now a programme of hospital closure, scheduled to be completed by 2005 and forming a major plank of 'The Same as You', the Scottish Executive's review of services for people with a learning disability. As institutions have closed, and people with learning disability take on a higher profile within society, it has become clear that, in two areas at least, the legal framework available was leaving many disabled people without appropriate legal protection. These were:

a) A lack of protection, both for the individual with a learning disability/incapacity and the person acting on their behalf in the matter of the individual's financial affairs, when they were not subject to either a curatory/power of attorney relationship or a patient in a hospital where managers were given powers to manage their financial affairs. Curatorys cost money and are, therefore, not applicable to those with only state benefits to manage; power of attorney requires that the person granting it is capable at the time, clearly not applicable to the majority of people with a learning disability who may need help to manage their financial affairs.

b) No legal means of consenting to medical treatment on behalf of an adult who was incapable of giving informed consent themselves without recourse to costly proceedings through the courts. Prior to this act, the only way in which another adult, whether it be parent, sibling, carer or other appropriate person, could legally consent to any medical intervention on behalf of the incapable adult was by means of a little used and known piece of Scots law dating back to the 1920s and enabling the appointment of a 'tutor dative'. The usage of this piece of legislation had increased during the latter parts of the twentieth century, but it was regarded as an outdated law and, importantly, was not subject to any external review. In addition, it involved expensive and time consuming applications to the courts and was regarded as a rather heavy handed means of consenting to treatment, which was clearly in the best interests of the individual concerned.

Parents and family carers had long felt it anomalous that they could not legally consent to medical treatment on behalf of their learning disabled offspring, particularly where there is a severe degree of learning disability. The age at which people are deemed adults and autonomous in terms of such decision making is set at 16 years, and the law took no account of the capacity of the individual. In many situations, the issue of consent was ignored and treatment given, including operative treatment, on the agreement of the parents or next of kin or, in the case of patients in a hospital, by the doctor responsible for them. This was all done with the best of intentions, but as the medical world became increasingly litigious, the doctors became more unwilling to act outwith the law, despite it (more often than not) being in the best interests of the patient. This resulted in some unnecessary delays in treatment for patients and more anxiety and worry for relatives at times of transition from children's to adult services.

The 'Adults with Incapacity (Scotland) Act 2000' became the first piece of legislation passed by the new Scottish Parliament. The purpose of the Act is to provide for decisions to be made on behalf of adults, who lack legal capacity to do so themselves because of mental disorder or inability to communicate. The decisions concerned may be about the adult's property or financial affairs, or about their personal welfare, including medical treatment. It is the first piece of legislation that brings together in one act, the two constituent parts of the framework that developed in the late nineteenth century with the passing of the 'Idiots Act', as noted in the introduction. It provides additional safeguards and supports for people who are incapable, but does not completely remove the necessity for people to be included in the provisions of the Mental Health Act, if necessary. However, all the guardianship provisions formally within the Mental Health (Scotland) Act 1984 are subsumed in this act.

The principles that are stated in the act are broadly as follows:

- Any intervention/decision must be of benefit to the adult
- The intervention should be the least restrictive 'consistent with the purpose of the intervention'
- Encourage the use of remaining capacity
- Take account of the views of the adult, if known, the nearest relative and primary carers, as well as any guardian or other legally appointed person.

It also makes it clear that the issue of capacity is not an all or nothing concept; people may have capacity in some areas and not in others. Incapacity is defined as incapable of:

- Acting, or
- Making decisions, or
- Communicating decisions, or
- Understanding decisions, or
- Retaining the memory of decisions.

By reason of mental disorder or inability to communicate because of physical disability.

So the legislation is aimed at people with learning disability, as well as those with other forms of mental disorder, including dementia, and those whose physical disabilities are such that they are unable to communicate in any meaningful way. Augmentation or assistance with communication is expected where appropriate, so an inability to speak does not of itself lead to the person being declared incapable. The assessment of capacity has to be made by a doctor and also has to be assessed in relation the specific intervention proposed. Therefore, incapacity in relation to financial affairs does not automatically imply incapacity in relation to personal welfare or consent to medical treatment. The Act covers:

- Attorneys with welfare and financial powers
- Access to funds held on behalf of an adult with incapacity
- Authority for hospital and care home managers to manage their finances
- A statutory authority for medical practitioners and those acting under their instructions to give treatment to adults with incapacity and undertake research in certain circumstances
- Welfare and financial intervention orders and guardianship.

For people with a learning disability, it is most likely that all except the first point above will be of relevance. Applications for welfare or financial interventions orders, or guardianship have to go before the court and require reports, in relation to the proposal, from two medical practitioners. One of these must be a specialist in mental disorder. For welfare interventions or guardianship applications, there must also be a report from a mental health officer (a specialist social worker). The orders are also tailored to meet individual need. They are not all or nothing arrangements as this would be inconsistent with the stated principles of the Act. A welfare guardian can be given the power to consent to medical treatment on behalf of the adult. There are appeal mechanisms and arrangements for regular review and oversight by appropriate bodies. A new office of 'Public Guardian' has been established to:

- Supervise guardians and those authorised by intervention orders
- Maintain a register of all documents relating to this and to continuing and welfare attorneys and authorisations to intromit (manage people's money)
- Investigate complaints relating to any of the above
- Investigate circumstances where the financial affairs of the adult appear to be at risk
- Provide information and advice.

In addition, the Mental Welfare Commission has responsibilities in relation to any of the areas of intervention where the adult is suffering from mental disorder.

Consent to medical treatment (Part 5)

As noted above, one of the main drivers for this piece of legislation was the lack of a straightforward legally valid means of consenting to medical treatment for people who, by reason of mental disorder, were unable to consent to physical medical treatment. In theory, this included issues, such as being prescribed and given two paracetamol for a headache. The Act requires medical practitioners who are treating incapable adults to complete a certificate stating that:

- The adult is incapable
- The treatment is necessary; and
- They have consulted all relevant parties.

The certificates, which can last up to a year, cover 'fundamental healthcare procedures'; these are treatments to which all adults are entitled, including nutrition, hydration, skin care, relief of pain, mobility, etc, and specific, longer term treatments, such as might be necessary for chronic physical illnesses. Any new illness that may require treatment is subject to a new certificate. The scope of the certificate would be delineated by a treatment plan attached to it, particularly where the individual had multiple or complex needs. In general, the person's general practitioner would be the appropriate individual to complete such a certificate, with additional 'one off' certificates provided by other medical staff, such as surgeons, as required. The certificates covering fundamental health care procedures, etc, are not meant to include those interventions that would normally require the signed consent of the adult. The certificates are also required to legitimise the treatments provided by other healthcare professionals, with the agreement of the person's general practitioner. So, physiotherapists, dentists, speech and language therapists, and clinical psychologists, for example, all require to have their inputs legalised by the certificate.

While the principles and intentions of the new Act have been welcomed, general practitioners and other medical staff are finding that the adherence to the guidelines is causing an increasing amount of work in an already stretched service. There are concerns about the competence of general practitioners in relation to the assessment of capacity in people with a learning disability, although not so much in relation to the elderly who may be dementing. It is also important to note that, in those circumstances where a welfare guardian has been appointed **and** they have been granted the authority to consent to medical treatment on behalf of the individual, then the general authority to treat under part 5 of the Act is not applicable, unless the doctor has been unable to contact the guardian to ascertain the position, and the treatment is in the best interests of the person concerned.

There is one important caveat to this; neither the GP, who signs a certificate, or a welfare guardian, who consents to treatment being given, has the power to authorise the admission of the person concerned to a psychiatric hospital against their will. Here the provisions of any mental health legislation would require to be utilised.

In England and Wales, there has been no separate legislation to clarify the law on consent and incapacity in relation to medical treatment. Instead, they have relied on common law provisions and the 'best interests' principles. The House of Lords has suggested that any action taken 'to preserve the life, health or well being' of a patient will be in their best interests. The best interests principle has also been held to be far wider than 'medical best interests' and to include welfare considerations. Therefore, assistance with dressing, washing and the consumption of food are all deemed to be in the individual's best interests. It has also been made clear that no health professional or relative/carer should sign a consent form on behalf of the individual; instead, the incapacity in relation to consent to treatment should be noted in the medical record. It will be interesting to hear whether doctors and others in hospital desist from asking relatives or involved healthcare professionals to sign consent forms.

For some treatments, it is still essential to obtain the consent of the courts. These are:

- Sterilisation for the purposes of contraception
- Donation of tissue, such as bone marrow
- Withdrawal of nutrition and hydration from a patient in a persistent vegetative state
- In situations where there is doubt as to the person's capacity or best interests.

Only time will tell whether the promise of the Adults with Incapacity (Scotland) Act will be fulfilled. It has been introduced in phases, part 5 commencing on 1st July 2002 and the final constituent part, governing the management of finances by care home managers, will become effective from October 2003 not April as previously thought. It remains to be seen whether the current pressure from GPs regarding the time consuming nature of the procedures laid down in the accompanying guidance notes will result in any modifications.

European Convention on Human Rights (ECHR)

The final piece of legislation, which merits mention, is that of ECHR. There are, of course, many other statutes that have a bearing on the lives of people with a learning disability. However, this is an important piece of legislation that has taken almost half a century to be included in British statute.

The European Convention on Human Rights (ECHR) was drawn up in 1950 and ratified by the UK in 1951. However, the Convention rights were not binding on either the devolved Scottish parliament or the UK parliament until the Scotland Act 1998 and the Human Rights Act 2000 came into force. Prior to this, the only recourse British citizens had was to take their case to Strasbourg and the European Court of Human Rights. It is now possible to enforce Convention rights in domestic courts.

The Convention rights likely to have the most impact on people with a learning disability are:

- The right to life
- Freedom from torture and inhuman or degrading treatment and punishment
- The right to liberty and security of person
- The right to respect for private and family life, home and correspondence
- Freedom of thought, conscience and religion
- Freedom of expression
- Freedom of assembly and association
- The right to marry and found a family
- The right to education
- The right not to be subjected to the death penalty.

There are, of course, other rights in the convention, and the interested reader is referred to the Human Rights Act 2000 and the ECHR itself for more detail. Most of the rights are not absolute and governments can place limitations on many of them in the interest of national security, the prevention of crime or the protection of health, morals, and the rights and freedoms of others.

The effect of all this is that any new legislation or Act of Parliament has to be compatible with the provisions of ECHR. This has implications for the new Mental Health Acts in both Scotland and England and, potentially, will lead to a large number of legal challenges to the enforcement of any such legislation. It is still not clear to what extent there will be successful challenges utilising the ECHR grounds. There have been a large number of challenges since 1999, most unsuccessful. Nevertheless, it is an area of the law that will be defined by case-law and, as the act now covers 'public bodies', there is potential for any acts by these bodies or people acting in a public capacity to be challenged. This includes health and social work bodies, as well as local councils, the police, etc.

As noted above, there are many other pieces of legislation that impact on the lives of people with a learning disability. It is an evolving picture, one which becomes ever more complex as power is devolved from centralised governments, on the one hand, and concentrated in multinational arrangements, such as the European Union, on the other. From the United Nations through to the Scottish Parliament, legislation is governed by overarching principles and shaped to fit local need. The lives of people with a learning disability are intimately affected by the interplay of the principles and societal need, nowhere more so than in the integration of health and social care.

References

The Human Rights Act (2000) HMSO, London

The Scotland Act (1998) HMSO, London

The Adults with Incapacity Act (2000) HMSO, Edinburgh

European Convention on Human Rights, as amended by Protocol No. 11, Directorate of Human Rights, Council of Europe, 1998

Mental Health Act (1983) HMSO, London

Mental Health (Scotland) Act (1984) HMSO, London

7
Integration: A Carer's Story

Jenny Whinnett

Behind labels, policy, legislation, strategy, and developments in thinking and attitudes are quite simply, real people; people we call 'people with learning disabilities'. People with learning disabilities are loved members of families, all of which have their own unique stories that will tell of heartache, joys, hopes and aspirations. Much is said and done in their name, and it is only recently that many have been enabled to tell their story. By listening to their stories and experiences, and moving away from seeking responses from services based on historical practice, needs of individuals and their families will be recognised.

This carer's story is significant as it focusses on a young man with profound and multiple learning disabilities. People with profound and multiple learning disabilities are frequently reliant upon their families and carers to tell their story and advocate on their behalf. The importance of good integrated care for people with learning disabilities and their families is highlighted in the story of Craig.

Early experiences

This is the story of Craig. We adopted Craig, who became a part of our family fourteen and a half years ago, a long, painfully thin scrap of humanity, who appeared to be able to cry at two levels; loud and ear splitting. How well we still remember walking round and round the lounge with Craig in our arms while attempting to appreciate Gene Kelly's 'Singing in the Rain' at 3.00am. We assumed all the crying in the early days to be due to his profound disability, but it is only in hindsight, and with seventeen years of fostering experience, that we now realise that Craig's distress at that time was due to the separation from his birth family. We received excellent support from the charitable fostering adoption agency, with which we worked, through their training programmes and regular social worker visits.

We were linked up to Craig's medical and therapeutic team within days of his arrival in our home, and his paediatrician at that time was the individual who gave us the most confidence in caring for someone with profound disability. He gave us very honest answers to our questions on Craig's prognosis, and treated us with respect at all times. The weekly visits to the child assessment centre to see the therapy team were vital to help me feel less isolated. I did not have the confidence to do anything with Craig unless the relevant therapist had given approval. It took a few weeks for me to remember that this was a baby boy who happened to have profound disabilities, and then overnight I relaxed and made a promise to him that he would have the best quality of life I could provide for him, full of experience. I enjoyed the contact with other mums at the centre, and was grateful for the advice from the therapists, but during those early years I felt so ignorant about my son's disabilities that I never had the confidence to give my views on subjects relating to his care.

Following the adoption, we had Craig's medical care transferred to our own local health authority. We were delighted when his paediatrician also took up a position within our area health authority to run their child assessment centre. Within a short time of taking up his position, he arranged a full week's assessment for Craig. We spent five days at the centre, where Craig had sessions with each member of the development team, and then, on the final day, they had a case conference, with every member of the team and my husband and myself attending. I had enjoyed the week up to this point, but we found the case conference very daunting, as there appeared to be many people sat round a table in a room, discussing my son. We wish we had been aware of the benefits of a citizen advocate then, as we would have greatly appreciated such support at that meeting. The outcome of the assessment on Craig was that the assessment centre could offer him one day a week in the support nursery. I transported him the seventy-mile round trip, and stayed with him during the day. He was allocated a one-to-one nursery nurse, and we had sessions with the therapy team. We also enjoyed access to the therapy pool when it was available, and sessions with the computer.

Leading to gastrostomy

Dduring his early years, Craig's health was affected by many chest infections, which resulted in frequent admissions to hospital. He had to endure blood tests and drips to ensure getting adequate fluids and drugs into him. The most serious illness occurred on a holiday trip to the island of Iona, when Craig developed a nasty herpes virus reaction, following contact with chicken pox. We had to dash across Scotland with a youngster who was deteriorating before our eyes. Craig was put onto a drip, and a nasal gastric tube for feeding. The dietician at the hospital during this admission was the first person to suggest that Craig may benefit from a gastrostomy, and I had the opportunity to see another little one who was already being fed via a 'Peg' tube. On Craig's return home, a number of appointments were made for Craig at the Children's Hospital, to investigate whether he was aspirating food and liquid into his lungs due to reflux, and his poor swallow reflex. Craig had to endure a 24-hour PH study, where a NG tube was inserted and attached to a monitor. How he hated the experience. Then followed the barium test. I administered the barium myself in an orange drink, and Craig appeared to have taken it really well, until we laid him down for the X-rays, and it immediately became apparent that Barium had entered his lungs. The situation was very serious, and professionals ran from everywhere. Craig still has flecks of Barium in his lungs to this day. We immediately requested an appointment with the surgeon who would perform the gastrostomy, and on our first visit, he stated that Craig would also require a fundoplication procedure to prevent the reflux that was clearly occurring. Craig's surgeon was very honest and clearly outlined the real risks to Craig of performing such major surgery.

My husband and I felt very nervous about making such a major decision on behalf of our son without being able to involve him. I eventually asked the surgeon for an honest answer to the question of whether, if Craig were his son, would he have this surgery performed on him. He answered, "Without hesitation." Craig was taken into the Children's hospital in the July of that year, so that he had the summer holidays to recover from the surgery. The day before his operation, we were shown the individual intensive therapy unit room with all the machines that would monitor Craig post operatively. We also met all the members of the team who would be caring for Craig, i.e. the gastrostomy nurse specialist, the dietician, anaesthetist, and nurses.

They would also be providing training to carers and myself who supported Craig's care. They trained me on the care of Craig's stoma, his feeding pump, and all the consumables he required to do with his feeds. Craig's operation was a terrifying experience. It was only supposed to take two hours, but eventually took six. The surgeon discovered that Craig had some of his organs in different places, and he also had very bad adhesions. It was the longest day of our lives. The surgeon was very sensitive and, as soon as he had completed the surgery, he came immediately to bring me up-to-date on Craig's situation. Following two days in the individual ITU, Craig had recovered well enough for him to be cared for in the four bed ITU, and he spent two weeks there recovering, while I learned about his future feeding requirements. The care and support that Craig and I received were excellent and, by the time we left hospital, I felt confident that I could cope with Craig's new feeding regime. I also had ongoing support from the specialist gastrostomy nurse through regular home visits and ongoing contact with the dietician.

Childhood health

Over the intervening years, and up to the onset of puberty, two years ago, Craig's health remained very good. He had to attend clinics for his orthosis, his wheelchair, his eyesight (during his early childhood), and orthopaedics. I have had a very good relationship with the professionals involved in Craig's care, but there have been isolated incidents that have left me shattered. On my first visit to the wheelchair clinic in my area, I attended the appointment on my own with Craig, as my physiotherapist had not been informed of the appointment. I was apprehensive, as I did not know what to expect. The therapists in attendance took lots of measurements, and then the consultant came into the room.

They started discussing different wheelchairs, completely ignoring Craig and myself, but I did realise from their deliberations that there could be a problem with the size of the car I had at that time. I was upset that they did not take into consideration the lifestyle that Craig lived with his family, and whether the wheelchair they were choosing would be suitable. I had the audacity to come into the discussion, and bring up our family lifestyle and the size of the family vehicle. The consultant exploded, and loudly said that I was an ignorant mother, and I might as well go and sling Craig in a hammock for the rest of his life and accept the resulting contractures if I did not accept that they knew best. The fact that I did not know what contractures were at that time is beside the point. I was in shock, as no one had ever spoken to me like that in my adult life. Craig's physiotherapist was able to inform me on the procedure of how to make a formal complaint, and then mediated with the wheelchair clinic concerning his seating requirements. I never saw that consultant again.

My son had to attend the ophthalmology clinic during his early years, as they assessed his vision, and he received all the usual eye tests. We were aware that Craig did have some visual impairment, and we always tried to perform activities within his field of vision as advised by the professionals. However, we became aware during Craig's early years that he frequently dropped his head and appeared to look at things with his eyes upward. I mentioned this to a visiting consultant running a visual workshop that I attended, and he identified that Craig had peripheral vision, and was achieving the best vision he could by dropping his head, and raising his eyes. I certainly gained a great deal from that workshop, but Craig had been let down by the ophthalmology clinic, which failed to recognise his peripheral vision. However since then, he has had very good service from the visual impairment support services.

Puberty

All young people have to go through puberty, and Craig was no exception. We became aware that the hormones were having their effect. His voice deepened, and he took a large growth spurt, similar to all boys of his age; sadly, it has not been an easy experience for Craig. Two years ago, his seizure control began to deteriorate, and there followed months of hospital admissions where his consultants struggled to stabilise his seizures and his health. He suffered a breakdown of his fundoplication, which required major surgery to repair and, while he was in hospital, his consultant neurologist, 'The Prof', used his recovery period to assess and change his seizure medication in an attempt to improve his stability. He was a tremendous support to me, and treated Craig with great kindness and myself with respect. I will always have the utmost respect for this consultant, and believe that he will always have the respect of all the parents and little patients that he will care for in the future. How many consultants would sit with a parent and youngster beside their bedside throughout the night? 'Prof' kept a bedside vigil with myself when Craig suffered the most appalling withdrawal from the drugs used post-operatively, and he appeared to be in terrible pain. He sat with me and encouraged me to keep talking to Craig quietly through the night, but at the same time he was continually monitoring him to check his level of awareness, and seizure control. I would have had terrible difficulty getting through that night without him, as it was very distressing to see Craig in that state. 'The Prof's' move back to his own country is a sad loss to our hospital.

Over the following six months, Craig's seizure control continued to be problematic, and the powerful drugs that were given to him affected his heart rate or his breathing, and resulted in him having further health problems. He underwent withdrawal of a drug because of allergic reactions, and close monitoring of the affects of a replacement drug being introduced. During this dreadful period, Craig also suffered two dangerous bouts of pneumonia that left our family very depressed and upset. The second of these admissions for pneumonia was made a nightmare for our family by the actions of a senior consultant. The morning following his admission, the physiotherapist on call arrived on the ward to work on Craig. I was very relieved to see that it was the physiotherapist who had cared for Craig since he was a little boy, and she knew his body very well. I had been up most of the night, in the ward, giving him chest percussion and suctioning him, and I was relieved to have her support.

On returning to the ward after a break, I was greeted with the curtains drawn around my son's bed and informed that the consultant on duty had been called. He had never had Craig under his care. Two junior doctors accompanied him, and I was pleased to see that the physiotherapist was still with Craig. The staff nurse who was caring for Craig stood by the bed, as he had supported the physiotherapist, while she worked on Craig's chest. The first words the consultant greeted me with on approaching my son's bedside, was to ask if we, as a family, had discussed whether to have Craig ventilated, if his lungs collapsed. He stated that they could not ventilate him in our local hospital, and it would require a long journey to a suitable hospital. The likely result would be that Craig would be unable to breathe unaided, and would remain on ventilation. Did I think this was in his best interest?

I went into shock. He was talking in front of my son, who was hearing this conversation. I answered strongly that Craig was fighting, and I did not believe that he was as serious as was being implied. The staff nurse who had nursed Craig through his previous pneumonia also stated that Craig did not appear as unwell as his previous episode. It was suggested that I contacted the family to discuss our choices, and then he left the ward. This experience had a devastating effect on me that lasted for months, because the consultant handled the situation so badly. How dare he be so insensitive as to discuss such matters 'over the head' of my son. Ethical decisions, such as resuscitation and ventilation should be discussed in depth with the family of someone with profound disabilities, when it becomes apparent that the person's health is deteriorating sufficiently that such a decision may have to be made, and it can be discussed in an atmosphere of sensitivity, and with the patient's own consultant. My son's consultant came to see my husband and I the following day, following our family discussion. He did concur with the other consultant's diagnosis that Craig would be unable to come off ventilation in such circumstances, but he definitely stated that Craig was recovering, and in no immediate danger of collapse.

Later that year, due to Craig's continuing health difficulties, a large meeting was convened to discuss his health issues, and what extra support could be put in place in the home, to minimise hospital admissions. Anaesthetists were present, along with many other professionals involved with Craig's healthcare, to give information, and ask what support they could give to Craig. My husband and I had previously discussed with Craig's citizen advocate and his social worker further support that we felt would benefit him and us, to enable him to remain cared for long term in his own home. We were also linked up with the community children's nurses, who work from the Children's Hospital, and support children with high health needs in the community. They have become a wonderful source of support to our family, but why have we only just been offered and received their input when we were in a period of so much stress? Their support would have been appreciated from the moment Craig came into our care. They have done a large amount of work in setting up two nights a week of overnight care for Craig in the home, and also overseeing the full training of all Craig's carers, in all aspects of his care. I have been fully involved in the training courses for the carers, and in the physical training pack that we have developed for all those involved in Craig's day-to-day care. I am delighted with the results, as all Craig's carers have the confidence to care for him when he is well, and when he may be unwell with his seizures or chest problems. This will result in fewer admissions to hospital, which is usually an ordeal for Craig and for us all as a family.

Caring for Craig in adult services

The hospital does not have the facilities for people with Craig's level of physical needs, so it is very difficult to toilet or bathe him. There is only one hoist in the hospital, so if it is required by another ward, it means that the nursing staff or me has to physically lift my teenage son, who is now as tall as his mum. The nursing staff are very helpful and caring, but there are never enough on duty to enable adequate support for Craig, so I never leave my son in hospital on his own. Nurses and doctors are not trained in the needs of someone with profound disabilities, so that is another reason for me to always remain with my son. I have often had junior doctors and nurses not recognise when seizures are occurring or how poorly Craig is feeling. Hospitals should all have specialist nurses who can support the staff and doctors with patients who have a learning disability, and profound disabilities, and all doctors should have some experience of learning disability and profound disabilities during their training. I look to Craig's medical care with some trepidation once he has to move on to the adult resources. There appears to be no consultants who specialise in the care of adults with profound disabilities, so Craig will have a succession of consultants in the different relevant disciplines. I do not believe that any one of them will really get to know my son as intimately as his present consultant, because they will see him less frequently, and only in their own speciality. I am concerned that this can have a bearing on the quality of care that Craig will receive as an adult patient. I am also very concerned that Craig will not receive the various therapies he may require in the future, and which he receives at present on a regular basis at his school from the community care team, led by his community paediatrician. I would like the reassurance that an adult community care team will continue the therapy input to Craig once he attends his adult resource centre.

Education choices

When Craig began to attend the child assessment centre in our local authority on a weekly basis, it quickly became apparent that one day a week was not enough input for Craig. I did not know what was available in the locality where I lived that would prove suitable for Craig, so I decided the best avenue would be to visit my local education offices, and find out what resources might be available to Craig immediately and to obtain information on his future education. I was given an appointment with an educational psychologist, and was very pleased with that first introduction to the world of Special Education. I was given an appointment immediately with the headmistress of the local SEN school and details of a local kindergarten in my own village that would be appropriate for Craig from the age of three years.

Pre-school experiences

I joined the local mother and toddler group, as this gave Craig the valuable opportunity of mixing with the village children, and I also enjoyed the opportunity to be with other mums. Craig thoroughly enjoyed the experience, accepting being climbed over while lying on his little wedge, or the wails of a toddler in a 'paddy'. The children also saw Craig as just another little boy, and the mums within the group accepted Craig for the lovely little boy he was. He was invited to all the outings and birthday parties, and always had a smile on his face at every new experience. The headmistress of the local SEN school also gave me valuable support during Craig's toddler years, by allowing me access to the school's therapy pool and a personal session of work with Craig on a weekly morning basis. I really enjoyed taking Craig to the school's 'day care' room (as it was called at that time) and joining in, with Craig, in the activities that were taking place with older children who also had profound disabilities. The class was led by a very dedicated lady, but there was no teacher working in the room. I saw a lot of sensory activities being done with the children, and they were all treated with respect, and physically cared for very well. The headmistress had recently been on a course using special teaching techniques for young children with profound disabilities that broke a task down into simple steps. Over a period of time, I worked with the headmistress using this technique making small advances with Craig's development. Craig enjoyed the experience, as he loved being in the classroom setting, and the use of the therapy pool. I did realise, though, that the facilities within the school were very limited for the pupils with profound disabilities.

Craig began at the local kindergarten following his third birthday. I was fortunate in knowing the staff very well, and I had done some preparation before I took Craig on a regular basis. At first Craig and I had made some short visits, so that we had the opportunity to get used to the environment and experience briefly some of the activities the children shared. Craig was the only child with disabilities on the two mornings he attended, but that did not prevent him from joining in the activities, or the imaginary play. The other youngsters accepted Craig totally. He always had the birthday candle placed on the table of his day chair, for the birthday child to blow out. Craig loved this responsibility. The children enjoyed turn taking in moving his arms and legs in the 'Action' songs, and he was always the train-driver or pilot of the aeroplane in the 'imaginary' playtime. The other children's mums were equally supportive, and asked for advice on what they could bring for Craig's snack when it was their turn to make elevenses, and he was always asked to the local children's parties. Craig loved the mornings spent at the kindergarten, and it really developed his ability to socialise with people. The kindergarten was run on a set routine, which was very beneficial to Craig, and it offered a set number of activities, so that the children developed their skills, as well as their social abilities. I remained with Craig during his time at kindergarten, but I was happy to develop this role and became a qualified kindergarten assistant.

Schooling

Following Craig's third birthday my educational psychologist held a meeting at the child assessment centre, and informed me that a 'record of needs' was being opened for Craig. We discussed all his therapeutic needs and what we, as Craig's parents, would wish to be included in the document. I had been given a small leaflet giving information on the record of needs, and asked the educational psychologist about a 'named person' for Craig. I was informed that my husband and I were articulate enough; therefore she did not believe one was required. I have since registered Craig's citizen advocate as his named person, and I am sorry that I did not have her included from the beginning.

Craig's choice of school was also discussed at the meeting, and it was suggested that we might benefit from viewing a school that was farther away from our home, but specialised in the education of children with profound disabilities, and was attached to a hospital that cared for people with profound disabilities. The school was very impressive. There was a lovely friendly atmosphere throughout, and parents were made very welcome. At that time, the school benefited from the facilities that it shared with the hospital, including the use of respite on the children's ward for families of the youngsters in the school. We felt reassured by the pool of expertise that was available 'on site' to meet Craig's needs and, following our visit to the school, we enrolled Craig. He started at the school two days a week, and for the first month I transported him the seventy five-mile round trips, so that I could learn from the teacher, and the therapists. He went up to the children's ward at lunch times, so that he could have a rest in a cot provided for him, and he had a nurse who fed and changed him. He continued part time at school, and continued his involvement with the kindergarten until he reached his first dentition at six years old. We had a very close relationship with Craig's school for the next ten years. I would frequently go and spend a day in the classroom, so that I could keep up-to-date on the work they were doing with Craig. They had yearly reviews of Craig's record of needs, and formal parents meetings.

While he was very young, he spent his days in a very therapeutic classroom, with a lot of sensory activities being offered, and they also concentrated on his developing physical needs. When he reached ten years old, he was moved into a classroom with older and slightly more able children. They were more vocal, and the environment was far noisier than his previous room. I was understandably anxious about how Craig would cope with all the young ladies he spent his days with (five teenage girls, and only one other boy), and all those monthly hormones. I should not have worried. Following the initial shock to his hearing, he took all the girls in his stride, and made a great pal of the other young lad in his class. He quickly adjusted to the new environment, and really enjoyed the new activities it offered. His new class teacher had immense specialist knowledge, and she began to concentrate on Craig's communication skills, and computer work. Craig spent three very happy years within that class environment.

The city education authority informed parents of children being educated in their special schools that they were looking at all their establishments. They were planning to rationalise, leaving only two specialist schools, and that most children would be transferred to learning support units attached to mainstream schools. We discussed our options for Craig at his annual review, and it was suggested that my husband and I should visit the specialist school within our own local authority and closer to our home. The head teacher was the same person who had given me so much support in Craig's early life, and she had not lost any of her enthusiasm. The school offered Craig a very good range of educational opportunities, with a highly skilled teacher in charge of the class in which Craig would be placed. The dynamics of the class were different to the one he had been used to, with two younger mobile children, but I recognised that Craig would enjoy the lively atmosphere that would produce.

Craig's health had become problematic, due to the onset of puberty, and we believed that he would benefit from the reduction in the time spent travelling to the local special school.

I put in writing to the local educational authority exactly what would be required to make it feasible for Craig to access his education at the local special educational school, including equipment and a one-to-one classroom assistant. I waited until I had official agreement to my requests before I put in our official proposal to transfer schools. I thought that I had covered every avenue, but during the last two years there have been a number of teething problems for Craig within his new school.

The first morning, the incorrect transport arrived, with a vehicle that Craig's wheelchair would not fit into, so we had to transport him ourselves for a number of days. We had to keep him off school for two days because there was no one to give him his daytime feeds, despite the gastrostomy nurse specialist having performed training within the school. Craig and the other youngster with profound disability had to be changed behind curtains in the quiet corner within the classroom for a number of weeks, because the alterations to the toileting area had not been completed during the holiday period. I became aware that the class was struggling with the physical care of my son, because on a couple of occasions I discovered that his personal care had been neglected due to the lack of support cover. I reasoned that if his personal care was not up to standard, then how could he be receiving the support he needed to access his education within the dynamics of that classroom. I quickly contacted my educational psychologist, and put in writing my concerns about staffing within Craig's classroom, emphasising that I did not want staff being pulled out of other classes to supplement Craig's class, but that permanent extra staffing hours required to be allocated.

I dealt with all of the initial difficulties that we encountered during the first year in Craig's new school through his educational psychologist, who was very supportive. I had to take the problem of the class alterations to the director of special education, because I was so disappointed that Craig's dignity was being compromised.

In spite of the problems encountered during the last two years within his new school, and even though he has had to miss a lot of schooling due to the serious health difficulties he has suffered, Craig has settled into his new school extremely well. He really looks forward to going to school every day, and gives a big smile whenever those who are involved within his school life are mentioned.

Future needs review

When children who hold a record of needs reach their fourteenth year, a special annual review is then held. The purpose of this review is to look at their post secondary school options, and to plan for that time. We had been thinking about this special review for some time, and I had been in discussions with Craig's citizen advocate, his social worker, and other relevant people. Craig's citizen advocate and I had taken the opportunity to visit the local day centre, to meet the warden, and view what facilities they could offer Craig in the future. Craig's social worker and myself had spent some considerable time producing an in depth document on Craig's future needs, and a 'wish list'. On the day of his future needs review, I discovered that he had been allocated only forty minutes. There was a brief discussion on Craig's education for the previous year, which had been very limited due to his poor health. There was a short discussion on how he would be linked up to the local day centre, and transferred to the adult care team, and that was that. There was no discussion around the large document that had been produced by myself and the social worker, or mention of our 'wish list'. Has the document been 'filed in the bucket'? Will anything come of the issues raised in it, or the 'wish list'? Our major concern for Craig's future is that he is going to disappear into the transition's 'black hole'. We wish to see a smooth transfer from local paediatric, and educational services, into adult resources; well planned, and properly resourced.

Social and leisure activities

Craig is a real 'party animal', if he is given the opportunity. He loves socialising and is a real people person, although he does not like it if a person speaks over his head as if he is not there. The purpose of our decision to foster teenagers was to give him the opportunity to have other young people around him and to lessen his isolation. People with profound disabilities are very isolated. Fostering has been a positive experience for all. Craig has enjoyed the company of the young people we have had in our care, and has become very close to one of our youngsters. Almost all the accommodated youngsters have gained from living with someone who has profound disabilities and seeing the problems they face in their everyday lives.

Craig loves outings, and will have a go at anything offered to him. We take him bowling and to the cinema on a regular basis, and he also has his favourite places, such as the Winter Gardens, and a local garden centre that also has an animal park. He loves the water, and I have found the most suitable pools for their water temperature and adequate changing facilities; however, they are fifty miles from our home. He especially enjoys a pool that has a wave machine. He might love the experience, but mum is nearly in a state of collapse hanging on to him while he is giggling being swished to and fro. I have taken Craig to a number of exhibitions and galleries, as he is naturally a very artistic young man; and, although physical access to buildings is slowly improving, changing facilities are the biggest bar to a normal social life for anyone with profound disabilities. Finding a toilet is something most people take for granted, but finding suitable toileting facilities for my son is usually impossible. I've lost count of the number of dubious, cold, damp toilet floors that I have had to lay my precious, vulnerable, son on, with only a blanket between him and the floor. On most occasions when we are travelling or visiting venues today, I change my son in the rear of our adapted minibus, as we have 'blacked-out' windows. Preferable to a toilet floor, but who should need to accept such conditions?

We have never let Craig's physical difficulties, or the blocks society puts on his lifestyle, prevent us from fulfilling our promise to Craig to give him a life full of experience. He has visited many parts of this country and overseas. Craig loves his holidays, and we have taken him on a number of pilgrimages over the years to the island of Iona, where we have enjoyed living with the community at the Abbey. It is quite a journey. Across Scotland, with two ferry crossings, and single-track road journey across Mull, but we all love the tranquillity and community spirit offered to the visitors there.

While serving as a Royal Marine, my eldest son fell in love with a young lady from Boston, USA. Due to Craig's many health needs, our visit to attend their wedding had to be planned with military precision. Craig thoroughly enjoyed the adventure. He played his role as the 'ring bearer' beautifully, and my daughter-in-law always says she has two husbands, because Craig said his vows along with his brother. On returning to Britain, we all required a couple of days to recover from 'jet-lag', but not Craig; he was just fine.

One of the most important events in Craig's life that he takes a full part in, is being 'Uncle Craig' to his nieces and nephew. Three years ago, Craig and I travelled down to Aylesbury to visit family, as a new baby was due. We made our way to the hospital; however, by the time we arrived, the new baby had arrived by an emergency caesarean. Thankfully, mum and baby were fine and Craig an uncle. He was thrilled with his little niece, and never took his eyes off her, until a nurse came and told us that the wheelchair was a health risk and Craig would have to leave the ward. We promptly wheeled the baby's crib out of the ward, and into an anti room, followed by Craig, so that both had the opportunity to spend time together. What would the hospital have done with disabled parents? Taken their wheelchairs away from them while in the maternity ward? Despite such an attitude, Craig has developed a wonderful relationship with his little niece and she with him. Even though she now lives in Boston with her parents and, sadly, they have had so little time together, she will always ask to speak to her 'Uncle Craigy' on the 'phone. I have produced a special sensory story about the birth for Craig, so that it has become his special story, and allows him to relive a special memory.

Support networks

Throughout Craig's life, there have been times when Dave and I have wondered if we were making the correct decisions for our son. The difficulties were not so great in his early years, as he was physically smaller, and his health was less problematic, also we were younger, and fitter ourselves. It is also normal for parents to make decisions for their young child. This did not lessen the desperate need for relevant information and support that we required, faced with caring for someone with so many difficulties and such an unknown future. That support came into our family's life nine years ago, when the new co-ordinator for **PAMIS** (a voluntary organisation offering support to people with profound disabilities and their carers) came to my home and asked what did I need to make my caring role easier. I spent two hours with her, pouring out my problems and frustrations. Within a very short time, an invitation arrived in the post to a workshop on equipment and handling within the home. They offered a crèche, and help with transport if required. The workshop was wonderful. We were each given a binder full of information to take away with us, to refer to if required, and we shared the workshop with invited therapists who learned along with parents and carers. We developed a mutual understanding of our situations, and it has certainly helped me to develop my relationship with Craig's therapists over the years.

I have been very fortunate to have the opportunity to develop relevant caring skills, and to have gained access to a great deal of relevant information through the many workshops that **PAMIS** have produced for carers and professionals. They have also given parents and carers, such as myself, the opportunity to give mutual support, because we are given the chance to meet together. Only we know what it is like to care for someone with so many difficulties, and only we could laugh at some of the unusual situations in which we may find ourselves. I am also involved with some particular projects that **PAMIS** are developing, such as 'sensory stories', and the 'guide to the elaborate curriculum'. They also have lobbied vociferously for adequate changing facilities, and we have produced a very informative and eye-opening video, which we hope will have an effect on planners throughout the country.

It is very important that Dave and I should get a break, both physically and mentally. I was aware many years ago that there was little respite offered in our local authority, so I was happy to be involved with the steering group that investigated the extent of the need for a Crossroads care attendant scheme in our area. We have never looked back. I was the initial co-chairperson when it started up, and the scheme has developed very successfully over the last ten years. I have four wonderful carers who are all fully trained in Craig's care, and the scheme gives Dave and I the opportunity to go out for a meal, and two unbroken night's sleep a week. I am delighted that the initial hard work has resulted in a very successful respite scheme within our area.

Dave and I also greatly benefit from a weekend break once a month, when Craig is cared for at a Church of Scotland respite centre. They are very caring, and give Craig the opportunity to escape from mum and dad, and spend some social time with his friends. The only problem with most respite services are that, because there are so few available, you have to take what is offered, and there is no choice of dates. If you are lucky, you may get a family to swap when you have something important planned, but we tend to have to plan our adult social lives around Craig's respite breaks. We have to pay more expensive prices if we want a weekend break, because nothing can be done spontaneously. We are fortunate to have this resource, but there is no emergency respite in the area, so Dave and I must never fall ill at the same time, or both of us have an accident, because I do not know where they would place Craig for respite in those circumstances. It is a constant worry to us, and other carers.

Preparing Craig for school in the mornings used to be a time of utter chaos, and bedlam; however, peace descended in our household three years ago when I was given the support of two local home carers. They have been fully trained in all aspects of Craig's care, and are also on the team of carers that do the twice-weekly sleepovers. They are very adaptable, and have become a very important part of our family support. It is quite innovative for home carers to have had the level of training that these willing people have agreed to attain, and I am very pleased that the home care service has agreed to the training for the staff.

Shortly after the finalising of Craig's adoption, the Charitable Fostering Agency offered us their newly formed advocacy service. They had made a commitment to all their young people and, although Craig was only very young at the time, they were happy to put him on the scheme. Over the next few years they kept his details up to date, but when the service went independent of the Agency the new co-ordinator visited my home and suggested that it was time to think of an independent citizen advocate for Craig. It didn't take me long to think of the right person, as she had lots of relevant experience, and she knew and cared for Craig a great deal. We were delighted when she agreed to accept the role, and she received the relevant training. We have been very grateful for her support over the past few years, as she has supported Craig at all his important meetings, and supported Dave and I when we have had to make important decisions. She is a very good friend to our family.

We are also fortunate to have the support of local carers support workers; although their remit is to support all carers, they are always there to talk to, and to try to get information if required. They will also mediate with other agencies if we need that support.

I hope that I have given a balanced view of our life with Craig; of the many highlights that we have shared with this sensitive and lovely young man, who we are so proud of, and who has brought us so much pleasure over the years. He has taught his family and the many people who have shared his life about tolerance, courage and, most of all, about keeping a sense of humour.

8

Integration and the Healthcheck 2000 Experience: Breaking through to better health for people with learning disabilities, in association with primary care

David Marshall, Gordon Moore and Roy McConkey

Meeting the health needs of people with learning disabilities

The health care of people with a learning disability has, in recent years, increasingly come under the spotlight. This interest has been accelerated by the changing emphasis in how care is provided. Historically, people with learning disability in need of care outside of the family, have been cared for in long-stay, institutionalised settings, staffed mainly by nurses. However, a major shift in such care provision has seen the reduction and closure of many of these traditional settings in favour of providing care in the community, thus having a major impact in the delivery of primary health care services for this client group.

Department of Health (1998), Howells (1996), Beange and Bauman (1991), and Wilson and Haire (1990) point out that the needs of people with learning disability living in community settings are not being recognised by primary healthcare services and are, therefore, largely unmet. Thornton (1997; 1996) argues that the awareness of the health care needs of adults with learning disabilities has tended to be limited within primary health care teams. Arguably, this could also be the case for people living in social care services, with staff who have little training or experience of health issues.

The following publications by the Department of Health have highlighted the subject:

- **The Health of the Nation**: a strategy for people with learning difficulties (Department of Health, 1995) points to the lack of attention previously paid to people with a learning disability in the area of health. The document emphasises that people with a learning disability are entitled to have equal access to all aspects of health promotion services, including: health education, health surveillance, and primary and secondary healthcare, with 'appropriate additional support as required to meet individual need' Department of Health, 1995)
- **The New NHS: Modern Dependable** (Department of Health, 1997) document gives direction to the many concerns, which have been raised in relation to service provision of the health care needs of the learning disability population and its future organisation
- **The Once a Day** (Department of Health, 1999) report purposed to promote good practice in enabling people with learning disabilities to access and receive good quality services from primary health care teams, and it refers to findings that people with learning disability 'access primary care much less than they need to'. This was substantiated in the Mencap Report 'Prescription for Change' (Singh, 1997), which states that 'on average, they (people with learning disabilities) made fewer visits to their GP than the rest of the population'
- **Signposts for Success** (Department of Health, 1998) has assisted in taking the process forward, by providing new guidance and information upon which to base good practice in relation to local health improvement programmes, to ensure that people with learning disabilities get the best from the NHS. This document highlights the importance of commissioning and increasing the accessibility of primary care services for people with learning disability, based on findings by the Department of Health that people with

learning disability 'visit their doctor less frequently than the national average'

- The Government's white paper on **'Valuing People; A New Strategy for Learning Disability for the 21st Century'** (Department of Health, 2001) highlights the fact that the most important issue, which the NHS needs to address on behalf of people with learning disabilities, is developing its capacity and skills to meet the identified health care needs. 'The health needs of people with learning disabilities may not be recognised by doctors or care staff, who have no experience of working with people suffering from difficulties in communication. Health outcomes for people with learning disabilities fall short when compared with outcomes for the non-disabled population' Department of Health, 2001).

However, a study by Janicki *et al* (2002) appeared to show that health visits for people with a learning disability over the age of 40 years might not be very different from that of the general population and, in some cases, was of a lower frequency in relation to specific illnesses. This study looked at health characteristics and health services utilization in older adults with intellectual disability living in community residence. They obtained information on a large-scale cohort of adults with intellectual disability and aged over 40 years.

The sample size included 1371 adults drawn from a convenience sample of 1600 group home residents. The main finding showed that the majority of subjects were in good health. 'The frequency of cardiovascular, musculoskeletal and respiratory conditions, and sensory impairments increased with age, while neurological, endocrine and dermatological diseases did not.

Psychiatric and behavioural disorders declined with age. When frequencies of age-related organ system morbidity were compared to data from the National Health and Nutrition Evaluation Survey III, it was found that adults with intellectual disability had a lower overall reported frequency of cardiovascular risk factors, including hypertension and hyperlipidaemia, and late onset diabetes. This seems to contradict the previous findings. However, the study concludes by suggesting that either a cohort effect is operating or that there may be an under-recognition of selected risk factors and diseases (Janicki *et al*, 2002).

Irrespective of whether or not people with intellectual disabilities have or have not increased health needs, it would appear that they do not access primary health care services as frequently as the general population.

Changing primary care needs

Changes in the morbidity and mortality rates can be seen in the life expectancy of people with a learning disability, which has increased in line with that of the normal population (Kerr *et al*, 1996). However, despite such changes, Singh (1997) highlights that people with a learning disability still suffer, increasingly, from shortfalls in the provision of primary health care. Added to this is the changing pattern of social care, with the exodus of people with learning disability from large institutions to community facilities having the potential to be seen as an increasing burden on the workload of the GP and primary health care teams (Kerr *et al*, 1996). Yet an effective and efficient GP service is vital to meet these increasing health demands.

Kerr *et al* (1996) suggest that doctors are given limited training in how to devise specific strategies to overcome difficulties in consulting with people whose language is poor. This might also pertain to many other healthcare professionals. Fraser *et al* (1996) suggests that clinical terminology is also a barrier to the patient's appropriate understanding, while Barker and Howells (1990), Beange and Bauman (1990), Howells (1996), and Minihan *et al* (1993) cite poor communication skills on the part of primary care staff, and the clients themselves, further acting as barriers to receiving appropriate treatment and care.

Failure by carers—both family and paid carers—to recognise the need for health checks, or to seek appropriate medical attention when required could also be a factor in people with a learning disability receiving an inadequate service provision.

They may also make the presumption that poor health is part of their disability and that little can or should be done about it.

Lawrie (1995) highlights the potential for some carers to be reluctant to take clients to see their GP because of concerns about the manifestation and embarrassment of presenting challenging behaviours; and, while Large and Jenkins (1999) see that long surgery waiting times prove problematic, Beange (1996) refers to short consultation times reducing the ability to provide accurate history taking.

Mant (1994) highlights the concerns of general practitioners with respect to screening procedures, and their opposition to regular health checks for people with a learning disability on the grounds that, while GPs agree in general that the day-to-day health care of people with a learning disability is their responsibility, some do not recognise a responsibility for health checks as part of health promotion with this client group. This is emphasised by one GP's response in 'Prescription for Change' (Singh, 1997). When asked about the subject of health checks, the response was, *'It's a waste because I don't think you are promoting anybody's health. It's a negative aspect of health promotion, in a sense it does not alter mortality or morbidity. I treat health according to needs'*.

The 'NHS—Health For All?' report, produced by Mencap (1998), cites Singh (1997) who pointed to the difficulties in using the general practitioner service when GPs are reluctant to provide health checks for people with learning disability. This, he argues, leads to unmet health needs and he goes on to cite the lack of treatment for hypertension and cancers (Whitfield *et al*, 1996) and lack of reviews of medication (Langan *et al*, 1994).

Surveys by Barr *et al* (1999), Wilson and Haire (1990), and Howells (1986) report high levels of unrecognised morbidity, yet low levels of health promotion among people with learning disability living in the community and attending adult training centres. Thus regular health screening has the potential for maximising the detection and amelioration of potential chronic health and life-threatening disorders.

Howell (1996) reports that, as a result of health checks given to 151 people with a learning disability, 75% required, but lacked innovative treatments in health promotion. In all, 36 people had circulatory problems, 75 had problems relating to eyesight and 20 were registered as obese. These findings were reflected in a study by Coles (1986) of health care needs of a group of people with a learning disability, in that 66% required medical attention for unmet health needs, which included referral for obesity and visual acuity problems. Wilson and Haire (1990) describe how 80% of a similar sample population had untreated medical problems that needed attention. This included 29% who were obese.

It is clear from the literature, and in relation to embracing the principal of inclusion (Department of Health, 2001), that planned action needs to be undertaken in relation to meeting the needs of the current population with learning disability. It can also be seen that people with learning disability often lead unhealthy lifestyles and unnecessarily develop physical health problems that can be prevented, or at least the impact reduced, by health promotion activities. Regular health checks have been proposed as one way to deal with the shortcomings in identifying and meeting the general health needs of people with learning disability.

Martin (1999) identified that health check clinics can help provide valuable information to purchasers and commissioners on demography and needs, as well as clinical information to primary health care teams. Martin compared a variety of primary health care models for people with learning disabilities and stated that health checks utilised by community learning disability nurses were useful in that they:

- Helped to profile people with a learning disability
- Identify health needs
- Promote patient/carer involvement in care
- Allow for time and ease of service
- Provide a comprehensive health check.

He further stated that GP-led health checks were an enhancement to nurse-led health checks in the following areas:

- Identification of health needs

- Provision of a comprehensive health check
- Prescribing interventions
- Ensuring health needs are met.

Howells (1996) sees that the responsibility must lie with the learning disability services to create increased links with primary health care. This is in line with the Department of Health (1998) who pointed out that, 'where health checks are available… (they have) usually been achieved by primary care and specialist services planning and working together'

However, for people with learning disability, it is a fundamental right to have access to mainstream health services in the first instance, with referral on to specialist services as needed. These specialist services would include both specialist learning disability services and medical specialities as appropriate.

Healthcheck 2000

Healthcheck 2000 was the initiative of the Learning Disability Programme of Down Lisburn Health and Social Services Trust Learning Disability Programme in Northern Ireland. The Eastern Health and Social Services Board provided special monies for the duration of the two-year pilot project.

The aim of this current initiative was to develop an integrated and inclusive health check (surveillance) service that would lead to improved health care, health promotion, and overall health gain for people with a learning disability. In so doing, the project sought to develop the healthcare provision of the specialist learning disability programme, by encouraging improved communication and working links with primary health care services. This would assist in targeting current and future health care needs, and minimising present gaps in service delivery for people with a learning disability. Thus, the project would provide information as to how health care provision could be made fully accessible to people with learning disability.

At each health check clinic, a GP was present, together with a male and female nurse with learning disability training and who were employed (one full-time; one part-time) by the learning disability programme of the Trust. Two GPs were employed by the project on a sessional basis, each attending one of two clinics held weekly. The nurses attended all clinics.

Clinics were held in local and accessible venues. Adults were screened in a range of facilities, which included both residential and daycare provision, a college of further education, a small number in GP surgeries and some in their own home. The location was chosen on the basis of the most convenient access to clients.

- At each health check clinic up to six persons were seen for half an hour each on average
- A total of 398 adults with learning disability attended the health check clinics; 345 were in the age range 19–49 years old and 53 were in the age range 50+ years. It is noted that there may be an under representation of those adults who are over 50 years old
- Clients were seen on their own or accompanied by a carer who was a relative, or key worker if living in residential accommodation. In all, 342 clients were accompanied to the clinic. Of the remaining 56 who were not accompanied, it was obvious that they were of a higher ability with many of them living independently within the community.

GP Reactions

Prior to starting the project, a questionnaire was sent to all GPs in its catchment area, which sought to elicit information on the attitudes and opinions of GPs towards screening of this population.

In all 74 (50%) of questionnaires were returned. Nearly one quarter of respondents stated that they provided a specific health check for people with learning disabilities. However, the non-respondents may inflate these figures. If recalculated for the total number of GPs, then only 12% report providing health checks.

The GPs provided reasons as to why they did not provide services, which included: lack of time; lack of resources; hadn't thought about it; is too difficult to do everything; too many sub group of patients; it was not policy; lacked training; and some were sceptical of the value of routine health screens.

One in five GPs thought the proposed Healthcheck 2000 clinic would be **very** helpful; a further 60% that it would be helpful, but 19% rated it as not **very** helpful, not helpful, or unhelpful. Of those who thought the health check may be 'helpful', the reasons given were that it would discover health needs; it would see those patients not seen on a regular basis; a specialist health check may be more comprehensive and may uncover unaddressed needs, e.g. dental or eye problems.

Most of the GPs thought that such a service should be undertaken by a team experienced in learning disabilities. However, those with experience of, and interested in the pilot project undertaken, were more in favour of it being done in their own practice, in conjunction with the learning disability team or a specialist nurse.

It was decided to employ two GPs on a sessional basis to take part in the HealthCheck project. This would add to the credibility, detail and outcome of the health checks. Further they would provide information to assist bridge the gap in understanding the problems experienced by GPs in everyday practice, and their facilitation of care for people with learning disabilities. In addition to this, they would have a credible liaison role with those GPs who were known to be sceptical in relation to the idea of providing regular health checks for people who have a learning disability.

Pre-HealthCheck information

Each client/carer was sent a consent form prior to attending the clinic. In line with the Principle of Autonomy, described by Brown *et al* (1992: p60), where 'no person is there just for our convenience', respect for each individual was ensured. The clients and their carers had the opportunity to make an informed choice as to whether they wished to take up the appointment to attend the HealthCheck clinic or not.

The consent form included the following statements, which were to be completed as to whether they agreed or did not agree to:

- attend the clinic, which may or may include screening blood tests, if indicated
- information gained at the health check being shared with care staff as appropriate, which included a copy of the results being sent to the client's GP
- information gained being used anonymously for medical or other health and social services research.

Respect was given to a person's refusal to take part in any aspect of the health check process. In all, 22 clients chose not to have a health check and five clients chose not to follow up health promotion activities.

The appointment letter informed clients of the time, date and location of the clinic they were invited to attend. They were asked to bring the completed consent form, HealthCheck questionnaire and urine bottle with sample.

HealthCheck questionnaire

A questionnaire was developed and sent to each person prior to the HealthCheck 2000 clinic taking place. This assisted in gathering information of the person's health history in an attempt to build an individual health profile on each person. The information gathered, included:

- **Personal details**: name, date of birth, medical number, contact number, gender, carer details, GP details
- **Physical details**: approximate date of last visit to doctor, consultant psychiatrist, hospital doctors, optician, dentist, audiologist
- **Physical health problems**: (experienced or family history of) heart disease, high blood pressure, asthma, diabetes, thyroid problems, epilepsy, cancers, mental illness, or allergies

- **Medication details**: type and dosage of all prescribed medication that a person is taking
- **Exercise details**: type of, time spent in undertaking activity
- **Dietary details**: perception of weight, weight changes, foods taken
- **Female health**: cervical smear, breast screen, period details
- **Services received**: domiciliary, multidisciplinary, day care, general care.

The questionnaire was to be completed in partnership between the person with a learning disability and his/her carer.

Many hours were spent in the development of this questionnaire in order to elicit the most appropriate and meaningful data about the client's health needs. It was essential that the questionnaire could be easily understood by people with learning disability and their carers. 'Getting the language right is the most important part of creating accessible documents' (Moffatt, 1993). The project developed the questionnaire not only to elicit the information they required within the HealthCheck, but also to be an educative tool for the carers and the client, especially in relation to diet and exercise. Although other questionnaires were already published, none met the specific requirements of the HealthCheck 2000 project.

The HealthCheck 2000 clinic

At the beginning of each clinic, the nurse and GP discussed the information in the HealthCheck questionnaire with the person with learning disability and/or their carer as appropriate. This provided vital information and links in relation to understanding many of the client's assessed needs. Each clinic provided the following health checks:

- Heart and chest sound, eye health and hearing health were specifically completed by the GP, as the nurses are not trained to complete these tasks
- Weight and blood pressure

- Breast examination
- Testes examination
- Feet
- Cholesterol
- Glucose
- Blood (if appropriate)
- Full body check, i.e. checking the skin from head to toe for any abnormalities.

These checks were completed by either the GP or the nurse. In many instances, it was evident that familiarity with the community nurse gained co-operation more readily than the unfamiliarity of the GP.

The nurse completed the eyesight test and the hearing test. Each nurse had received training in eye testing technique. The Kay Picture Test, a series of pictures adapted to meet the necessary requirements for eye testing in cases where the client may not understand conventional formats, was used.

The hearing test was completed using a standardised audiometer test. This involved clients putting on a set of earphones. Tones of different pitches were played and the clients were expected to react or not react depending on whether they heard the tones or not.

Validity and reliability

The reliability of the clinical testing carried out by the project team was checked by repeating the tests. This repeat testing was carried out by two people, without conferring, within the one health check session, or as soon as possible after. This check compared the measurements taken by one health check doctor with another doctor; it compared the two nurses employed on the project, and the nurse ratings achieved on hearing and vision, with assessments made by an experienced speech and language therapist. This was done on assessments of 14 people.

Agreements for doctors ranged from 85% to 100% on ratings of blood pressure, chest and heart sounds, breast and testes examination, and eye and ear problems.

Similarly, the agreements between nurses ranged from 86% to 93% on skin, mobility, hair and feet problems. Agreements with a speech and language therapist on hearing was 91%, but lower (71%) on vision problems.

IT Database

A database for recording all the details of each person screened was developed by the project team in conjunction with the IM&T development team of the Trust. This was loaded onto a laptop, which could be easily transported to and from the different locations of the clinic. The HealthCheck team were able to record:

- clinical information elicited by HealthCheck questionnaires completed by the client/carer prior to the clinic
- clinical observations obtained by the project nurses and doctors at the clinic
- referral information relevant to GP and/or healthcare professional.

The database was able to print a standard pro forma listing the outcomes for action following the client's health check assessment.

The database had the potential to act as a future resource for streamlining report generation, as it collates information in one system. For example, the database could be programmed to find listings of clients by specific topics, such as, cardiovascular, sexual health, and mobility.

The query section had been set up to allow the project team to choose and 'run' queries on behalf of learning disability services within the Trust. However, this process happened infrequently, and it is questionable as to whether the enormous amount of time put into its development was appropriate. The database system has now been updated and this will allow for a clear communication process and evaluation analysis in the future.

Referrals following the HealthCheck

Clients and their relatives received a paper copy of the HealthCheck results to take away from the clinic. Carers were also advised of conditions that required early referral to a GP or support from other health care professionals. The detail of any referral information to specialist services was recorded on the information sheet. This included the name, address and contact number of the health care professional or service concerned.

The health care professionals to whom clients were referred were selected on the basis of their specialist practice and association with the learning disability services. An agreed referral listing was made prior to the clinic's commencement. Where a service did not take a direct referral, such referrals were channelled though the client's GP for action.

A paper copy of the results was also sent to the client's GP. Having been given this referral information, the onus was on the carer/person with learning disability to follow up the referral(s).

Results

The most commonly identified 'problems' in the health screens were overweight and obesity (64% persons); reduced vision (41%); foot problems (38%) and excess ear wax (30%). However, a wide range of other conditions were also identified. *Table 8.1* summarises the referrals made of adult persons following the health check. It is noted that some individuals had more than one referral to specific agencies. The bulk of referrals went to GPs, followed by health promotion and podiatry.

Table 8.1: Referrals of adult persons following the HealthCheck

Referral to	No	% of total	Examples of detected conditions
GP	298	(52)	Hypertension, varicose veins, ataxia, ear wax, menstrual problems, excema, diabetes, polycystic ovaries
Health promotion	111	(19)	Weight reduction, smoking cessation
Podiatrist	68	(12)	Damaged nails, fungal nails, corns, athletes foot
Optician	28	(5)	Poor visual acuity, reassessment of glasses, poor vision
Audiologist	20	(3.5)	Reduced hearing, hearing aid problems
Dentist	19	(3.3)	Dentures, oral hygiene
Consultant LD	9	(1.5)	Aggressive outbursts, calcium deficiency, choreathetosis
CNLD	5	(0.8)	Continence problems, random blood sugar, blood tests, personal hygiene, bereavement counselling
Others	15	(2.9)	Flat feet, underweight, raw area (buttocks), breast screen
TOTAL	**573**	**(100)**	

Referral to 'health promotion' constituted the name of the person being compiled on a list by the health check project nurses. This information then informed the project as to where to target health promotion activity. This took the form of Activate Health Promotion Classes—a programme of exercise, dietary and relaxation activities devised by the Health Promotion Agency in Northern Ireland and adapted by the Healthcheck 2000 project teams to meet the specific health promotion needs identified within the project.

(Full details of the results of the health screening can be had directly from the authors—Marshall D, McConkey R, Moore G, *Healthcheck 2000: Breaking through to better health for people with a learning disability;* Evaluation Report. C/o Mr Gordon Moore, Down Lisburn Health and Social Services Trust, Disability Resource Centre, Downshire Hospital, Ardglass Road, Downpatrick, Co Down, BT30 6RA, Northern Ireland.)

Health promotion

The health screening identified that over three in five adult people with learning disabilities (64%) were either overweight or obese (Marshall *et al*, 2003). People aged 40–49 years, who were obese or very obese, had raised blood pressure, which could dispose them to other health problems; e.g. strokes.

Some clients, who were identified from project results as being overweight, were offered health promotion classes. These clients formed a convenient sample, based in two day-care centres and one residential home.

The HealthCheck's nurses set up health promotion classes because no suitable classes were available. Neither the Health Promotion Section within Down Lisburn Trust or the primary care practices were able to organise these classes; however, the classes were to act as a model for others to follow, pending their successful outcome.

Twenty-five clients, who had been referred for weight reduction, took part in a series of health promotion programmes held at three different locations. Ten attended evening classes in a leisure centre, nine attended a day centre programme and six attended a group made up of residents from a residential facility. The classes included three elements of essential health promotion activity: exercise, healthy eating, and relaxation. An active health promotion package designed by the Health Promotion Agency in Northern Ireland was adapted to meet the assessed health promotion needs of clients seen at the clinics, with the information being given at an appropriate cognitive level.

The exercise programme included exercise to 'rap', which proved popular in that its repetitive lyrics were easily learned and retained.

The healthy eating activities were very diverse, from practical cookery sessions, to eating out, to making scrapbooks on healthy eating ideas.

The level of social interaction within the group was high. The group leader and staff had to think and talk about their lifestyle too, which encouraged the group. Some members of the group were more enthusiastic than others, while some needed a more individual approach. Full use of the leisure centre with the general public increased integration with leisure centre staff, and raised their awareness of the needs of this client group. The group mixed well with each other. Outings, which included a visit to the pub and bowling alley, displayed excellent group dynamics and social interaction at its best.

Communication skills were developed through interaction between the clients and those with whom they came into contact, such as, the staff at the leisure centre, in relation to paying for the ticket at leisure centre, asking for a racket and ball from the receptionist, listening during discussion group and giving their own point of view.

Only one client withdrew after the first class. Some were very keen, and others needed a little persuasion. Two clients initiated further evening classes through negotiation.

The classes did produce a significant weight loss for participants in a relatively short period. The 20 participants who had weight problem had a mean weight of 85kgs (SD 19.4) at the first session, but this had dropped significantly to 81.6 kgs (SD 17.8) over a six-week period ($t=4.6$ $p<0.000$). Likewise, the mean BMI score at the outset had been 33.5 (SD 5.9) and this fell to 31.9 (SD 5.4) ($t=5.26$ $p<0.000$). This meant that two people who had been overweight were now classed as 'normal'; one person moved from obese to overweight and three very obese people became 'obese'. However, it is not known whether these reductions were maintained. There were no significant differences in weight loss by gender, Downs's syndrome or age.

After the classes finished, staff were encouraged to incorporate this healthy lifestyle approach into aspects of daily living, e.g. walking to the day centre instead of using the bus, providing a well balanced diet. The healthy lifestyle approach was carried into other aspects of daily routine, i.e. shopping, cookery club and keep fit sessions (twice weekly).

Evaluation of the HealthCheck project

GP views

A second questionnaire was sent out to the 91 GPs who had been sent a referral letter regarding one of their patients: 70 (77%) replied. In all, 41% felt it had not created any extra work for them, 52% noted some extra work, while 7% said it created a lot of extra work. Likewise, 50% thought that any future screenings should be carried out jointly between their practice and the learning disability team, whereas 61% of those GPs who had not been sent a referral from the project, thought it would be better done by a specialist team compared to 20% of GPs who had a referral.

None of the doctors reported having received any postgraduate training in learning disability, which is consistent with research completed by Thornton (1996), showing that doctors had received a very low percentage of formal training in learning disabilities. However, 81% expressed an interest in having more training and 86% indicated that they would be willing to attend a structured training day. These results compare with those found by Singh (1997), who found that, in his research, 73% of his study sample of GPs said they would welcome more training for treating people with learning disabilities. Conflicting research, by Murdoch (1984), showed that doctors expressed mainly negative responses to the proposal of more training.

In being asked to rate the importance of having support from various specialists using a four part scale, from 'very unimportant' to 'very important', the greatest majority felt that community nurses for learning disability were rated as 'very important' in line with GPs, followed, in order, by social workers, psychologists, speech and language therapists, and consultant psychiatrists (for a fuller report, see McConkey *et al*, 2002).

Client/carer views

Following the health screens for adults, each client/carer was given a feedback questionnaire and a stamped addressed envelope. Of the 398 health checks carried out with adult persons, replies were received from 86 carers (22%). While this was a poor response, it is not untypical of postal surveys of carers. Almost all (94%) rated the service as being 'very helpful' or 'helpful' to the person with learning disabilities. Reasons for this, included: that it 'provided up-to-date information on health' and that the staff took time to listen and explain procedures'. Only 6% saw it as being 'unhelpful' or 'not very helpful'. Reasons for this were that 'explanations were too fast', or that 'explanations were not directed to the client'.

Similar responses were found when respondents were asked about the helpfulness of the service to them as carers. In all, 95% rated it as 'very helpful' or 'helpful', with only 5% noting it as 'unhelpful'. The reasons were not noted.

When asked their opinion as to where the health check might be best carried out, the most popular location was that of the Adult Training and Resource Centre (61%), where the advantages highlighted were: that it had familiar surroundings, it was handy/convenient, relaxed, attended daily with easy access, and time to discus any problems arising. The next most popular was the GP surgery (19%), followed by health clinics (15%), and own home (9%).

Opinion was also divided as to the frequency with which checks should be carried out. Around one-third (35%) thought they should be done annually, 19% once every two years and 44% once every three years. Only two people (2%) thought they did not need to be done. Those who responded as finding the HealthCheck 'very helpful' and 'helpful' would like it to be carried out at least once every three years, if not more frequently, and two-thirds felt it was best done in adult day centres.

Health care professional questionnaire

Questionnaires were sent to health care professionals of whom there were 31 to whom clients had been referred. Clients/carers were asked to access the appropriate health professional via their community nurse, social worker or directly themselves. However, this meant that not all health care professionals would have seen the referral if it had not been passed on.

Of these, six people felt screening should be done in the future by a team experienced in learning disability; 1 by a specialist nurse and nine by their own practice (i.e. three dentists, three opticians, two podiatrists and one clinical medical officer). The questionnaire did not ask about GP screening.

All the heath care personnel respondents felt that it had generated some extra work in the form of additional referrals, notably the podiatrist.

Only one of the 16 respondents had attended any form of structured postgraduate training in managing the health care of people with learning disability. However, the remaining 15 were all willing to attend a training day addressing aspects of learning disability care.

Lessons from the HealthCheck Project

It has been clearly shown that all people with learning disabilities, no matter how complex their needs, can have a health screen done in 'ordinary surroundings'. GPs and health care professionals welcome the screening service and there are indications that they would be prepared to become more involved with the provision of screening services. The project identified—yet again—that the key health issue for this group is 'overweight' and 'obesity'. It demonstrated that health promotion activities could have some impact on this issue when health promotion classes were developed to meet their needs. It also identified a small number of high-risk health problems in certain individuals, which could have been life threatening; problems, such as, testicular cancer, polysystic ovaries and undiagnosed diabetes.

What's the point of screening?

The end result of screening is to produce health gain in the designated population. For those with learning disabilities and additional needs, this is not an easy undertaking as both their biology and upbringing may be working against the attainment of good health. In recognition of this, a range of health service professionals are employed in this endeavour, including: GPs, health visitors, specialist doctors, specialist nurses, PAMS and so on.

It was noted from the literature that the health needs of people with learning disabilities could be easily overlooked and, hence, the role of providing a health check would be to bring their needs to the attention of the existing professionals. However, this argument has one fatal flaw; it presumes that the existing services will be able to attend to the problem and deliver the consequent 'health gain'.

Follow-up information from referrals was obtained through carers completing a postal questionnaire for each referral that had been made. A high response (86% of referred 'problems') was obtained to this request for feed back. However, only two of the 70 referrals for weight reduction reported any weight loss. This data raises crucial questions. Do they imply that little that can be done about the problems identified; were the necessary services not available; could carers not access them, or were they unwilling to access them? These questions are central to any health gain strategy.

Obviously, in a time-limited project, it is unreasonable to expect to see demonstrable health gains, especially as feedback on referrals was sought soon after people had been screened. However, had the project been rooted more in existing services, would this issue have arisen to the same extent? It was evident that the focus of health checks must shift from identifying problems to ensuring that systems and 'treatments' exist to deal with these problems.

Was the population screened, a representative sample?

The vast majority of the screens were undertaken in day centres and residences (90.3%), with only 9.7% done in health centres (35), or through home visits (4). Hence, the procedures developed by the project may be more appropriate for use in certain settings and more suited to being undertaken by dedicated screening personnel.

It was evident from the known statistics that a sizeable number of people who did not use or attend these services did not get a health screen, and age or ability comparisons were unable to be made. It is likely that those who were not screened tended to make less use of services and were aged over 50 years. If that is so, the data obtained may underestimate the health problems that are more likely to occur with age. Evenhuis *et al* (2001) highlights this point in discussing how the health status and health needs of adults with learning disabilities change, as they get older. Janicki *et al* (2002) refer to how numerous commentators have noted that many age associated conditions and diseases go undetected among community-dwelling adults with intellectual disability because of a lack of awareness among primary carers or clinicians, deficient or non existent screening practices, or a lack of focus on health surveillance in general (Allen *et al*, 1999; Carslen *et al*, 1994; Evenhuis *et al*, 2000; Harper and Wadsworth, 1992). This reflected the general finding of the Healthcheck 2000 project as opposed to Janicki *et al*'s (2002) suggestion that health for people with a LD (over the age of 40 years) might not be very different from that of the general population.

Moreover, to ensure a complete representative sample, it is recognised that modified procedures may be needed in contacting and screening these groups, from those used by HealthCheck 2000.

Is a specialist screening service needed?

HealthCheck 2000 was set up as a specialist service within the Trust's learning disability programme, and trained learning disability nurses were employed by the project. This can be justified in various ways; for example, in terms of expertise needed to interact with these clients; familiarity with the service systems involved with these clients; and having the skills to detect potential health problems.

The most commonly identified 'problems' in the health screens were overweight and obesity; vision problems; foot problems, and excess ear wax. This raises the issue as to whether or not carers were aware of these problems and, if so, what actions if any they had taken to resolve them? What would encourage carers to undertake regular health checks and what training would they need to identify problems of this sort?

By contrast, specialist procedures were used to detect other problems, although the incidence of these were low; for example, blood and urine tests; breast and testes examination; heart and chest sounds. However, these are all within the competence of GPs and practice nurses. Indeed, the increased willingness of GPs to become involved in health screening found in the second survey may derive from an awareness that this falls within their areas of competence and expertise.

The project staff noted that the only aspects of the health screening that required specialist learning disability expertise was their knowledge and understanding of learning disability and in managing the process. The main difficulties they noted were: taking bloods, physical examinations—especially with people who had autism—undressing and weighing people who had difficulty in standing. They also noted that communication is easier when you are familiar with this client group (both doctors had prior experience) and that it is helpful to have a knowledge of individual communication systems for certain clients. It is suggested that these skills could easily be acquired by interested primary health personnel through setting up teaching/awareness sessions, which could be delivered by either a learning disability nurse and/or a speech and language therapist. Encouragingly, 81% of GPs expressed an interest in further training.

Following on from the HealthCheck Project, Down Lisburn Trust, through the use of community learning disability nurses working in collaboration with primary care, is now providing health checks that are undertaken by GPs and practice nurses, and which involve other members of the primary care team.

Over a period of time, the learning disability nurses would withdraw from these clinics as competency is gained in meeting the communication needs of clients in relation to understanding their health needs. The community learning disability nurse would then act in an advisory capacity or in an 'on call' basis where specialist assistance is required.

Can the health of people with learning disabilities be improved?

In broad terms, the increased life expectancy of these people suggests that the answer is 'Yes'. However, this may result more from better treatment when people become ill, rather than an emphasis on health promotion. The issue of cost-benefits comes into play. It is argued that early detection means less costly tertiary care in acute hospitals; also less dependency in residential settings, e.g. supported living rather than nursing home care. As Singh (1997) highlights from his study, a sizable percentage of GPs did not agree that people with a learning disability should receive a regular health check and, if they were to, this would have funding implications in relation to GP payments. Within the HealthCheck 2000 study, one GP highlighted the current financial conflict that he would have in sustaining regular health checks without appropriate additional funding; he had a large learning disability nursing home within his practice.

The data on obesity is especially concerning. This suggests that exercise and diet must be a focus of attention from a young age and effective means found for preventing weight problems developing, as it appears that the prognosis for dealing with them when it becomes established is not particularly good.

Problems with hearing and vision also need to be addressed, as they occur with much higher frequency than they do in the general population, as do problems with feet. This may necessitate greater education of carers and improved access to key services, alongside a much stronger emphasis on health promotion in the job description and role of workers within learning disability services—both day and residential.

Conclusions

We draw the following conclusions from our experiences on the HealthCheck project:

- A specialist health screening service is not needed for people with learning disability. Rather, it should be the responsibility of primary care personnel (GPs, practice nurses) with assistance, at least initially, from staff from learning disability services—most likely community learning disability nurses. Their linkage would help to establish the screening procedures in GP practices and their ongoing input may be needed, particularly with clients who have additional needs, such as, multiple disabilities or challenging behaviours
- Training opportunities should be made available to interested GPs and practice nurses. Within practices, one partner might take particular responsibility for dealing with this client group. This practice has been initiated by one GP practice partnership in North and West Belfast, whereby one GP has taken a lead responsibility for overseeing GP provision for people with a learning disability. A specialist practice nurse assists in this initiative. However, it is of note that there is a large learning disability population within the practice catchments area, which may justify such an undertaking and commitment of resources. The possibility of GPs holding clinics in venues, such as day centres, could also be considered
- The materials developed by the project could be used or adapted by primary care personnel for use in their practices. For example, the computer-based recording systems could be incorporated into GP databases
- The job description of all specialist workers in learning disability services should emphasis their role in health surveillance and promotion. This is especially so for workers in

residential services in both the statutory and independent sector. Training modules on these topics should be available to all staff and they should be encouraged to be suitable role models for their clients

- The health needs of people with learning disabilities aged over 50 years should receive particular attention. The older persons screening schemes used with the general population should be offered at age 50 years to those with learning disabilities
- Mainstream health promotion services have a particular role to play in equipping staff in disability services to become more proactive and effective health promoters.

  Carers need to be informed about the role they can play in identifying potential health problems and in reducing their risk of occurring. Booklets and video programmes on topics, such as obesity, should be prepared for use within training courses and events for family carers, domiciliary staff, and staff in specialist services
- Future research should focus on determining effective means of encouraging weight loss, the prevention of foot disorders, and reducing the impact of sensorial impairments
- Screening for overweight/obesity in children should be targeted early, with suitable health promotion/dietary advice and exercise programmes implemented to reduce the incidence of obesity or related illnesses (hypertension, CHD) in later life
- Suitable tailored programmes of exercise and activity should be used with children/adults to promote healthy lifestyles especially in day centres and residences.

References

Allen M van, Fung J, Jurenka SB (1999) Health care concerns and guidelines for adults with Down syndrome. *Am J Med Gen* **89**: 100–10

Barker M, Howells G (1990) *The Medical Needs of Adults: Primary Care for People with a Mental Handicap*. Occasional Paper 47. Royal College of General Practitioners, London

Barr O, Gilgunn J, Kane T, Moore G (1999) Health Screening for people with learning disabilities by a community learning disability service in Northern Ireland. *J Adv Nurs* **29**: 1482–91

Beange HP (1996) Caring for a vulnerable population. *Med J Aus* **164**: 159–60

Beange H, Bauman A (1991) Health Care for the developmentally disabled: is it necessary? In: Fraser W, ed. *Key Issues in Mental Retardation Research*. Routledge, London

Beange H, Bauman A (1990) Caring for the developmentally disabled in the community. *Aus Fam Phys* **19**: 1558–63

Brown JM, Kitson AL, McKnight TJ (1992) *Challenges in Caring: Explorations in Nursing and Ethics*. Chapman and Hall, London

Carlsen WR, Galliuzzi KE, Forman LF, Cavalieri TA (1994) Comprehensive geriatric assessment: applications for community residing, elderly people with mental retardation/developmental disabilities. *Men Retard* **32**: 334–40

Cole O (1986) Medical screening of adults at social education centres whose responsibility. *Ment Handicap* **14**(6): 54–56

Department of Health (2001) *Valuing People: A New Strategy for Learning Disability for the 21st Century*. HMSO, London.

Department of Health (1999) *Once a Day—One or more People with Learning Disabilities are Likely to be in Contact with Your Primary Healthcare Team. How can You Help Them*? HMSO, London

Department of Health (1998) *Signposts for Success in Commissioning and Providing Health Services for People with Learning Disabilities*. HMSO, London

Department of Health (1997) *The New NHS: Modern, Dependable*. HMSO, London

Department of Health (1995) *Health of the Nation. A Strategy for People with Learning Difficulties*. HMSO, London

Evenhuis H, Henderson CM, Beange H, Lennox N, Chicoine B (2001) Healthy ageing—adults with intellectual disabilities; physical health issues. *J App Res Intellect Dis* **14**: 175–94

Evenhuis H, Henderson CM, Beange H, Lennox N, Chicoine B, and Working Group (2000) *Healthy Ageing—Adults with Intellectual Disabilities; Physical Health Issues*. World Health Organization, Geneva

Fraser W, Thomas P, Duckworth M, Joyce J (1996) Clinician's limitations with describing communication. By our frames we are hung. In: Muir N, ed. *Communication with the Mentally Ill Patient*. Kingsley Press, London

Harper DC, Wadsworth JS (1992) Improving health care communication for persons with mental retardation. *Pub Health Rep* **107**: 297–302

Howells G (1996) Situations vacant: doctors required to provide care for people with learning disability. *Br J Gen Pract* **46**: 56–60

Howells G (1986) Are the medical needs of the mentally handicapped being met? *J Roy Coll Gen Pract* **36**: 449–53

Janicki MP, Davidson PW, Henderson CM, *et al* (2002) Health characteristics and health services utilization in older adults with intellectual disability living in community residences. *J Intellect Disabil Res* **40**(4): 287–98

Kerr M, Dunstan F, Thapar A (1996) Attitudes of general practitioners to people with learning disability. *Br J Gen Pract* **46**: 92–94

Langan J, Whitfield M, Russell O (1994) Paid and unpaid carers: the role in and satisfaction with primary care for people with learning disabilities. *Health Soc Care* **2**: 357–65

Large J, Jenkins L (1999) Don't overlook a special group of patients. *Pract Nurse* **17**(3): 178–81

Lawrie K (1995) Better health for people with learning disabilities. *Nurs Times* **91**(19): 32–34

Mant D (1994) Editorial: Health checks-time to check out? *Br J Gen Pract* **44**: 51–52

Marshall D, McConkey R, Moore G (2003) Obesity in people with learning disability: The impact of nurse-led health screenings and health promotion activites. *J Adv Nurs* **41**(2): 147–53

Marshall D, McConkey R, Moore G (2000) *HealthCheck 2000, Breaking Through to Better Health for People with a Learning Disability. Evaluation Report*. Down and Lisburn Health and Social Services Trust, N Ireland

Martin DM (1999) A comparative view of primary health care models for people with learning disabilities: Towards the provision of seamless health care. *Br J Learn Disabil* **27**: 58–63

McConkey R, Moore G, Marshhall D (2002) Changes in the attitudes of GPs to health screening of patients with learning disabilities. *J Learn Disabil* **6**(4): 373–84

Mencap (1998) *The NHS-Health for All*? Mencap, London

Minihan PM, Dean DH, Lyons CM (1993) Managing the care of patients with mental retardation: a survey of physicians. *Ment Retard* **31**: 239–46

Moffatt V (1993) *A Guide to Creating Accessible Documents for People with Learning Disabilities*. Southwark INFORM Publication; National Disability Information Project, Southwark, England

Murdoch JC (1984) Experiences of the mothers of Down's syndrome and spina bifida children on going home from hospital in Scotland 1971–1981. *J Ment Defic Res* **28**: 123–27

Singh P (1997) *Prescription for Change*. Mencap, London

Thornton C (1997) Meeting the health care needs of people with learning disabilities. *Nurs Times* **93**(20): 52–54

Thornton C (1996) A focus group enquiry into the perceptions of primary health care teams and the provision of primary health care for adults with a learning disability living in the community. *J Adv Nurs* **23**: 1168–76

Whitfield M, Langan J, Russell O (1996) Assessing general practitioners care of adult patients with a learning disability; case control study. *Q Health Care* **5**(1): 31–35

Wilson DN, Haire A (1990) Health care services for people with a mental handicap living in the community. *Br Med J* **301**(6765): 1379

9
Integrated health care for people with learning disabilities

Craig Melville, Jillian Morrison, Linda Allan and Juliet MacArthur

Many people and organisations contribute to the development of health and the delivery of health services. The quality, speed and responsiveness of the journey is determined by how effectively these different people and organisations work together ... it is not just the NHS which provides health care services. Local authorities, voluntary organisations, independent providers and community health groups all have key roles to play.

Our National Health (Scottish Executive, 2000a)

Introduction

In order to deliver high quality, low risk and cost-effective services, models of health care systems are a constant focus of public policy across the world. Therefore, most major political institutions devote considerable resources to examining the challenges incumbent in providing quality health care. The quote above introduces the reasoning behind the recent policy shifts towards models that place an emphasis upon greater integration and collaboration across and within groups. Although these developments are at an early stage, intuitively, it is difficult to argue with the proposals. This chapter will describe what is known about the health needs of people with learning disabilities, and some of the shortcomings of existing services. The policy context and theory behind integrated care will be described before considering its implications on the provision of services for people with learning disabilities. Several examples of innovations that represent a shift towards greater integration of services will be used as illustrations.

The health needs context

The number of people in the United Kingdom with a learning disability has increased over the last 40 years. This increase is estimated at 1.2% a year since 1960, and will continue to grow by over 1% a year for the next ten years. An increase in older people with a learning disability has also been reported (McGrother *et al*, 2001). In the mid 1960s, some people with a learning disability were cared for in hospitals, although the majority have always lived within the community. By the late 1990s, this number had decreased by approximately 75%. This significant decrease in inpatient care, and an increase in life expectancy, have raised demands for generic primary and secondary health care services, as well as community-based, specialist services for people with a learning disability.

The health needs of people with learning disabilities have been divided into three categories (see *Box 9.1*). There is a strong evidence base for a high level of health need among people with learning disabilities (Beange *et al*, 1995; Cooper 1997; 1998; Espie and Brown, 1998; Royal College of General Practitioners, 1990). These studies show that, when compared with the general population, adults with learning disabilities have a higher level of physical and mental health needs. This finding is thought to be due to the influence of biological, developmental and genetic factors, adverse experiences or disadvantages in early life, and limited social opportunities. Despite these high levels of health need, people with learning disabilities have been found to consult their general practitioner (GP) less often than other people and have a higher level of unmet health need (Howells, 1996; Lennox and Kerr, 1997; Royal College of General Practitioners, 1990; Webb and Rogers, 1999; Whitfield and Russell, 1996; Wilson and Haire, 1990). There is a recognition that the significant barriers facing people with learning disabilities in accessing health services (Howells, 1996; Lennox and Kerr, 1997; Mencap, 1998) are contributing to their unmet health needs.

Box 9.1: Three levels of health needs of individuals with learning disabilities (Scottish Executive, 2002)

Everyday health needs	For example, the need to be registered with a GP, included within national health screening or health promotion programmes, and being able to access health care for problems that affect the whole population in a similar way; i.e. chronic disease management programmes
Extra needs because of learning disabilities	Many people with learning disabilities will require support to understand information, preparation and education for health care interventions. Additionally, some people with learning disabilities have health needs that are specifically associated with the underlying cause of their learning disability; e.g. adults with Down's syndrome require annual thyroid function tests
Complex health needs	People with learning disabilities who have complex health needs may have a wide range of health need that can co-exist; e.g. poorly controlled epilepsy with multiple seizure types, mental health problems, dementia, challenging behaviour, autistic spectrum disorders, sensory impairments, feeding problems, and multiple physical disabilities

A suggested solution is the development of one of a range of possible health screening programmes for people with learning disabilities (Lennox *et al*, 2001; Martin *et al*, 1997; Martin and Roy, 1999; Webb and Rogers, 1999). Such a programme would help to identify unmet health needs. However, to subsequently meet these needs would still require the strategic redesign of services.

The Health of the Nation: A Strategy for People with a Learning Disability (Department of Health, 1995) highlighted that people with a learning disability were part of the community, and that there was a need for society to become more responsive to their healthcare needs. It was more recently reported that there remains a need for solutions to address the changes in demographics and epidemiology of people with learning disabilities (Department of Health, 2001).

Within government, the needs of people with learning disabilities have been reviewed, with The Scottish Executive and the Department of Health undertaking a national review of services (Department of Health 2001; Scottish Executive, 2000c), highlighting the importance of accessible services, partnership working, and greater integration of services for people with complex health needs.

Therefore, the high levels of unmet health needs and the need to improve the accessibility of services have been recognised on several levels. A key question is whether greater integration of health care services will address these issues. The critical measure must be whether the changes and developments improve health *outcomes* for people with learning disabilities. To fully appreciate the move towards integration of services, it is important to understand and consider the broader context of health care policy, in addition to the policy influences on service development that are specific to learning disabilities.

The context of integrated health care

The importance of systematically considering care systems was emphasised in the World Health Report 2000, *Health Systems: Improving Performance* (World Health Organization, 2000). At a regional level, the World Health Organization (WHO) European Office for Integrated Health Care Services was set up to 'encourage and facilitate changes in health care services in order to promote health and improve management and patient satisfaction by working for quality, accessibility, cost-effectiveness and participation' (WHO, 2001). Although recognising that services will vary in different geopolitical areas, it is argued that some key components of integration that improve outcomes and quality of care can be identified and then used to inform the development of effective services.

At a national level, the integration of care services has increasingly been an important policy objective. The development of models of care that support greater integration of health and social care systems has initially focussed on community care for older people, but the principles and proposals, with the emphasis on partnership working, is now being applied across the public sector, including those with a focus on people with learning disabilities. For example, within Scotland there is support for care services, through the work of the Joint Futures Unit (see www.scotland.gov.uk/health/jointfutureunit). Like the World Health Organization (WHO, 1999), it is now recognised that a lead role played by primary care is developing integrated care services (Scottish Executive, 2000a; Scottish Office, 1997). Furthermore, there is an emphasis on the importance of making primary care more accessible (Scottish Executive, 2001). This recognition of the need to refocus and redesign health systems has brought about the subsequent changes that are being interpreted and implemented by national governments. These shifts in policy have led to several innovations in the provision of health care services that will be described later. In order to view these in context, a general description of the theory and conceptual basis of integrated care is given.

The conceptual basis of integrated health care

A general definition of integration is, '*...the act of making a whole out of parts; the co-ordination of different activities to ensure harmonious functioning...*'. More specific to care systems, '*Integrated care is a concept bringing together inputs, delivery, management and organisation of services related to diagnosis, treatment, care, rehabilitation and health promotion. Integration is a means to improve the services in relation to access, quality, user satisfaction and efficiency*' (WHO European Office for Integrated Health Care Services, 2001).

Health care provision involves large, complex systems. These generally include multiple, separate, but interconnected parts, which are required to co-operate and collaborate to accomplish defined tasks. Within such complex systems, there is scope for problems, such as poor communication or duplication of assessments, to affect patient outcomes and cost-effectiveness. An example of such a complex health care system is the five-tiered model of health care illustrated in *Box 9.2*.

Box 9.2: The five-tiered model of health care (Scottish Executive, 2002)

Tier 0	**Community, public health and strategic approaches to care** The promotion of the general health and well-being of all people with learning disabilities in all settings in the community. This includes public health and specialist nurses working with communities and local services to promote involvement, social inclusion and raise awareness of health issues
Tier 1	**Primary care and directly accessed health services** Access for all people with learning disabilities to primary care services and directly accessed health services, such as: community pharmacy, dental and optician services
Tier 2	**Health services accessed via primary care** These services work in support of primary care services in meeting general and additional health needs by providing appropriate assessment, treatment and specialist advice. Such services include: outpatient, domiciliary and inpatient services delivered from general hospital services, and palliative care
Tier 3	**Specialist locality health services** Focusses on specialist learning disability/mental health/child health services that are provided on a locality basis. These services work to support primary care services and others providing advice, assessment, interventions and treatments for specialist learning disability health needs. Specialists provide advice and practical support to people with learning disabilities, their families, and to local authority or voluntary sector providers, such as: schools, day services and short break services
Tier 4	**Specialist area health services** These consist of highly specialist area and regional services. They might be special assessment and treatment inpatient units, or area-wide specialist additional support teams for people with complex challenging needs, or forensic services for people with learning disabilities. Might be inpatient as well as in-reach models

Given the recognition of the wider context of health for people with learning disabilities, additional dimensions need to be considered. It is inevitable that people's social circumstances impact upon their health and well-being. For example, an individual with a learning disability, living in a community where he/she has no access to employment, structured daytime activities, or leisure facilities, is at risk of obesity, depression and other health problems. Therefore, as stated in the quote that opens this chapter, health care provision is not solely the responsibility of the NHS. It is important to consider and actively involve social work, housing departments, voluntary organisations, and representatives from carer and service user groups in the planning and delivery of integrated services.

Within such a framework, **horizontal integration** describes the bringing together of professions and organisations that operate within the same tier in the care model. An example is joint working in multidisciplinary community teams. **Vertical integration** involves bringing together services operating in different tiers, as in having trained learning disability professionals working in a primary care setting.

In theory, the greater integration of care holds several benefits:

- Improved clinical outcomes
- Greater cost-effectiveness
- User and carer involvement
- Improved communication.

Despite these putative advantages, and their intuitive appeal, both horizontal and vertical integration contain significant challenges for those involved. Both of these forms of integration require partnership working. However, a distinction has been made between co-operative partnerships and co-ordinating partnerships (Perri *et al*, 1999). Unless the factors that are central to facilitating inter-professional collaboration (see *Box 9.3*) are addressed, there is a danger that partnerships will remain at the lower co-operative level and fail to develop fully.

Table 9.3: Some aspects of partnership working (adapted from Perri *et al*, 1999 and Henwood and Hudson, 2000)

Key components in achieving interprofessional collaboration include:

- A common language, facilitating clear communication and sharing of knowledge
- A shared set of values, objectives and clear definitions of respective roles in carrying out relevant tasks
- A respect for the autonomy of those from different professional backgrounds

These factors will influence which of the two types of partnership are set up:

- **Co-operative partnerships** are characterised by enlightened self-interest. Partners pursue their own goals by co-operating with others. There is a low level of trust and maintaining the partnership requires minimum time and effort. The focus on more superficial issues produces short-term solutions
- **Co-ordinating partnerships** have a shared vision underpinned by common values. There is a mutual trust and a deeper understanding of purpose. These facilitate effective, stable longer-term working patterns and improved outcomes.

There are various service designs that could be considered under the rubric of integrated care. In recent years, *seamless care, care management, integrated care pathways* and *managed clinical networks* are some of the terms that have been used. Whilst there is some overlap between some of these models, they remain distinct. One or another may be more appropriate in different geographical or clinical settings. However, as will be discussed later, with specific reference to services for people with learning disabilities, there has been little evaluative research of the costs and benefits of such models of care.

Integrated health care in learning disabilities

Specialist health care services for people with learning disabilities have been working examples of integration of services, for a considerable time prior to public policy moving in this direction. Community learning disability teams are examples of horizontal integration- with professionals from different backgrounds, or statuatory agencies, working together. Yet, the greater proportion of people with learning disabilities living in the community, recognition of the level of unmet health needs and the barriers to accessing appropriate services has necessitated consideration of new models of service provision. Some examples of integrated care will be considered as a means of considering the implications for service users, carers and service providers.

Examples of best practice in integrated care

Multi-agency joint working

In Scotland, the *Joint Futures* agenda has been extended from care of older people (Scottish Executive, 2000b) to include services for people with learning disabilities and mental health services. Although different types of relationships can exist between agencies and organisations (Woods and McCollam, 2002), current emphasis is on greater integration through the joint resourcing and joint management of merged services. In Glasgow, health services and social work services have formally moved towards this with the creation of the *Glasgow Learning Disability Partnership* (Glasgow Learning Disability Partnership, 2001). A single management structure, budget and shared assessments are central to the partnership that has adopted a care management model of service provision. People with learning disabilities will have their care needs assessed and flexible, individual packages will be provided to meet these identified needs. In terms of healthcare, the partnership has invested in greater integration and collaboration with Primary Care whilst maintaining specialist learning disabilities' health teams. In theory, this model should develop tier 0 and tier 1 services, while improving communication and collaboration between the services in different tiers. Therefore, it will be able to address the three types of health needs shown in figure 1 and could reduce the high levels of unmet health needs. Furthermore, the partnership working between professionals from health and social work backgrounds will be able to address the social issues that impact upon health, such as poverty, housing and employment.

Box 9.4: The Primary Care Liaison Team, Glasgow

The Primary Care Liaison Team (PCLT) is a two year funded project whose aim is to complete a comprehensive health check on every known adult who has a learning disability in the Greater Glasgow area and improve access to primary care services for people with learning disabilities. The team also has a remit to provide training to LHCC staff, general practitioners, district nurses, practice nurses and receptionists. The PCLT works within Greater Glasgow Primary Care Trust and is funded by Greater Glasgow Health Board. The PCLT includes:

- Learning disability nurses
- General practitioners who provide an effective link between geographical primary care services and specialist learning disability services
- The speech and language therapist produces information in an accessible format. An example is the handheld health record provided to clients after the health check
- A senior health promotion officer is producing a health promotion strategy for people with a learning disability in Glasgow and facilitates networks with stakeholders.

The team is committed to working in partnership with:

- The University of Glasgow to investigate the team's impact and interpret the health check results. Publication of the findings promotes the sharing of information and evidence-based practice
- Glasgow Healthy City Partnership, supporting the senior health promotion officer in promoting health and reducing health inequalities across Glasgow
- Users and carers whose involvement relies on good networks. They are consulted on aspects of service provision and training on values, attitudes and communication. Service users and carers are offered support to participate in providing training where they have shown a desire
- Voluntary and charitable organisations who act as stakeholders of the project, benefiting through sharing information and promoting effective working by pooling resources and experiences.

By working together with interested partners, it is hoped that, through publication of research findings, best practice can be replicated nationally and internationally.

Primary care services

Strategic policy has promoted a central role for primary care in integrated models (Scottish Executive, 2000a; WHO, 1999). This could hold particular benefits for people with learning disabilities, in that it may allow the design of services to address the high levels of unmet general health needs (Royal College of General Practitioners, 1990; Beange *et al*, 1995; Espie and Brown, 1998) and problems in accessing services (Howells, 1996; Lennox and Kerr, 1997; Mencap, 1998). One example of such a model is the Primary Care Liaison Team (PCLT), in Glasgow (*see Box 9.4*).

The Primary Care Liaison Team aims to increase inclusion by improving the health care opportunities available to adults with learning disabilities. This is achieved by education and training, the sharing of knowledge and raising awareness of the health needs of people, in tandem with a co-ordinated programme of health checks and plans of care. This model embraces both horizontal and vertical integration. Furthermore, the partnership with the University Affiliated Programme for Learning Disabilities of the University of Glasgow, ensures that the project is subject to careful evaluation. For example, the health check was evaluated in a pilot study before being rolled out and studies to examine the benefits to service users and service costs are ongoing.

Acute hospital care

Research into the experience of people with a learning disability using acute, general hospital services tends to reveal dissatisfaction with the care provided and expressions of negative associations, including fear, lack of understanding (Hart, 1998; 1999) and isolation (Barr, 1997). There are several examples, throughout the UK, that suggest greater integration more closely addresses the needs of people with learning disabilities accessing acute health care. Expanding networks are emerging allowing the sharing of good practice. The Access to Acute (A2A) Network is now well established throughout England, and is endorsed by the Foundation of Nursing Studies as a forum for sharing best practice for learning disability care in hospital services. A2A has recently collated examples of best practice (A2A, 2002), including:

- Learning disability liaison nurse working with the accident and emergency department, the surgical assessment ward, the central outpatients department and gynaecology wards in North Staffordshire

- Learning disability liaison service in Lothian that incorporates a liaison nurse protocols, flow charts and an assessment tool to identify additional care needs (further details outlined below)
- The Birmingham Specialist Trust team of nurses and support workers who provide a liaison service to six hospitals in Birmingham and district. Their role is to provide support to patients and training to hospital staff
- The Sheffield Teaching Hospital project that has led to the development of patient and carer audit tools, care pathways and standards, referral guidelines for GPs, pre-admission assessment questionnaires and close collaborative working with the community learning disability teams
- Pain clinics for people with a learning disability in North Derbyshire Trust.

The Lothian Model of Acute Hospital Liaison

Since its inception in 1998, the Lothian Learning Disabilities Project has led to the development of a range of initiatives designed to support patients with a learning disability, their carers and health care staff, in the delivery of appropriate health care. Some examples of joint working by Lothian Primary Care NHS Trust (LPCT) and Lothian University Hospitals NHS Trust (LUHT) include:

- Appointment of a whole time equivalent, learning disability liaison nurse based within the general hospital service. This post is funded by the primary care trust. The post holder provides both direct and indirect care to clients and their families, in hospital and in the community, as well as contributing to a range of education and training programmes within the LUHT
- Development of a joint protocol that outlines general principles and processes related to the care of patients admitted

electively, or as an emergency, to the acute hospital. The key elements of the protocol are summarised in a series of five flow charts that have been distributed to all wards and departments for adult services within the LUHT

- Formal links between the community learning disabilities teams and the practice research development and education unit (PRDE), of the LUHT
- An annual, collaborative seminar focussing on the care of people with learning disabilities in the acute hospital. This multi-professional forum attracts staff from both acute and primary care and, to date, the content has concentrated on the client's care journey, consent, and communication
- The Lothian Learning Disabilities Working Group, with representatives from PRDE, the Royal Hospital for Sick Children, the three clinical divisions and the social work department within LUHNT, the clinical service development management, the clinical development nurse within LPCT and two carer representatives.

An audit of carer satisfaction with the liaison service revealed that they value the support of the liaison nurse and feel that the service has improved their experience of acute hospital care, in comparison to previous experiences.

Integrated care pathways

Integrated care pathway (ICP) are tools that can be used to co-ordinate and monitor the care provided within complex integrated services. They are flexible and can be tailored for specific clinical settings or particular diseases. Furthermore, they allow agreed evidence-based standards of care to be set and monitored when considering clinical effectiveness. In a series of papers, the Birmingham Partnership for Developing Quality has described the development of three ICPs for the assessment and management of hearing impairment, epilepsy, and challenging behaviour (Ahmad *et al*, 2002a & b; Brady *et al*, 2002; Pitts *et al*, 2002; Ahmad *et al*, 2002) in people with learning disabilities. These illustrate the complexity and potential value of integrating services to address complex health needs.

The examples above are just some of the different models of greater integration in health care provision that can, potentially, improve aspects of the journey of care for people with learning disabilities. One other model, likely to emerge over the next years, is the managed clinical network (Scottish Executive, 1999). The concept of managed care stems from the United States of America and it is unclear how the concepts can be adapted to alternative models of health care provision. Nonetheless, managed clinical networks may offer some advantages in addressing complex health needs that require integration of services across several tiers (see *Box 9.2*). For example, there are proposals to develop managed clinical networks for autistic spectrum disorders or for epilepsy services.

Conclusions

Models of care that involve partnership working and greater integration of services are central to current developments across the public sector. These represent a significant change in working practices and present challenges to all stakeholders in the process. Even with a shared vision and a commitment, there are several potential barriers to taking this forward (Hardy *et al*, 1999). Regardless of whether these barriers are operating at an institutional, inter-professional, or individual level, studying the process of integrating services will provide opportunities to overcome them.

There is an increasing emphasis upon evidence-based practice in health care. Therefore, like the rest of the population, people with learning disabilities have a right to expect services that have been subjected to careful evaluation. With specific reference to the developments in health care for people with learning disabilities, there is no published research evidence on the impact of greater integration of services. This will be important to address, in order that the strengths and weaknesses of particular models can be identified and applied to future development of services. While the theories and concepts behind integrated care suggest considerable benefits to service users, robust evidence to demonstrate significant improvements in the quality of services, outcomes, or cost-effectiveness is awaited.

References

Access to Acute Network (A2A) (2002) *Good Practice Examples* Unpublished document.

Ahmad F, Bissaker S, de Luc K *et al* (2002a) Partnership for developing quality care pathway initiative for people with learning disabilities. Part i: Development. *J Integr Care Pathways* **6**: 9–12

Ahmad F, Bissaker S, de Luc K *et al* (2002b) Partnership for developing quality care pathway initiative for people with learning disabilities. Part iic: Epilepsy. *J Integr Care Pathways* **6**: 90–93

Barr O (1997) Care of people with learning disabilities in hospital. *Nurs Stand* **12**: 49–56

Beange H, McElduff A, Baker W (1995) Medical disorders of adults with mental retardation: population study. *Am J Ment Retard* **99**: 595–604

Brady S, Ahmad F, Bissake, S *et al* (2002) Partnership for developing quality care pathway initiative for people with learning disabilities. Part iia: Hearing impairment. *J Integr Care Pathways* **6**: 82–85

Cooper S-A (1998) A clinical study of the effects of age on the physical health of people with intellectual disabilities. *Am J Ment Retard* **102**: 582–89

Cooper S-A (1997) Epidemiology of psychiatric disorders in elderly compared with younger adults with learning disabilities. *Br J Psychiatry* **170**: 375–80

Department of Health (2001) *Valuing People: A New Strategy for Learning Disability For the 21st Century.* HMSO, London

Department of Health (1995) *Our National Health: A Strategy for People with Learning Disabilities.* HMSO, London

Espie C, Brown M (1998) Health needs and learning disabilities: an overview. *Health Bull* **56**: 603–11

Glasgow Learning Disability Partnership (2001) *The Development of Area Learning Disability Teams.* Glasgow

Hardy B, Mur-Veeman I, Steenbergen M, Wistow G (1999) Inter-agency services in England and the Netherlands: A comparative study of care development and delivery. *Health Policy* **48**: 87–105

Hart SL (1999) Meaningful choices: consent to treatment in general health care settings for people with learning disabilities. *J Learn Disabil Nurs Health Soc Care* **3**: 20–26

Hart SL (1998) Learning-disabled people's experience of general hospitals. *Br J Nurs* **7**: 470–77

Henwood M, Hudson B (2000) *Partnership and The NHS Plan: Cooperation or Coercion? The Implications for Social Care.* Nuffield Institute for Health, Leeds

Howells G (1996) Situations vacant: doctors required to provide care for people with learning disability. *Br J Gen Pract* **46**: 59–60

Lennox NG, Green M, Diggens J, Ugoni A (2001) Audit and comprehensive assessment programme in the primary healthcare of adults with intellectual disability: a pilot study. *J Intellect Disabil Res* **45**: 226–32

Lennox NG, Kerr MP (1997) Review: primary health care and people with an intellectual disability: the evidence base. *J Intellect Disabil Res* **41**: 365–72

Martin DM, Roy A (1999) A comparative review of primary health care models for people with learning disabilities: towards the provision of seamless health care. *Br J Learn Disabil* **27**: 58–63

Martin DM, Roy A, Wells MB (1997) Health gain through health checks: improving access to primary health care for people with intellectual disability. *J Intellect Disabil Res* **41**: 401–408

McGrother C, Thorp C, Taub N, Machado P (2001) Prevalence, disability and need in adults with severe learning disability. *Tizard Learn Disabil Rev* **6**: 4–13

Mencap (1998) *The NHS—Health for All? People with Learning Disabilities and Health Care.* Mencap National Centre, London

Perri T, Leat D, Seltzer K, Stoker G (1999) *Governing In The Round. Strategies for Holistic Government*. Demos, London

Pitts J, Ahmad F, Bissaker S *et al* (2002) Partnership for developing quality care pathway initiative for people with learning disabilities. Part iib: Challenging behaviour. *J Integr Care Pathways* **6**: 86–89

Royal College of General Practitioners Working Party (1990) *Primary Care for People with a Mental Handicap: Occasional Paper 47.* RCGP, London

Scottish Executive (2002) *Promoting Health, Supporting Inclusion: The National Review of the Contribution of All Nurses and Midwives to the Care and Support of People with Learning Disabilities.* The Stationery Office, Edinburgh

Scottish Executive (2001) *Access to Primary Care Services in Scotland.* The Stationery Office, Edinburgh

Scottish Executive (2000a) *Our National Health: A Plan for Action: A Plan for Change.* The Stationery Office, Edinburgh

Scottish Executive (2000b) *Community Care: A Joint Future.* The Stationery Office, Edinburgh

Scottish Executive (2000c) *The Same As You? A Review of Services for People with Learning Disabilities.* The Stationery Office, Edinburgh

Scottish Executive (1999) *Introduction to Managed Clinical Networks in Scotland.* Management Executive Letter, MEL (99) 10, St. Andrew's House, Edinburgh

Scottish Office (1997) *Designed to Care.* The Stationery Office, Edinburgh

Webb OJ, Rogers L (1999) Health screening for people with intellectual disability: the New Zealand experience. *J Intellect Disabil Res* **43**: 497–503

Whitfield ML, Russell O (1996) Assessing general practitioners' care of adult patients with learning disabilities: case control study. *Q Health Care* **5**: 31–35

WHO European office for integrated health care services (2001) *Integrated Care: Working Definition*. WHO, Barcelona

Wilson DN, Haire A (1990) Health care screening for people with mental handicap living in the community. *Br Med J* **301**: 1379–81

Woods K, McCollam A (2002) Progress in the development of integrated mental health care in Scotland. *Int J Integr Care* **2**; available at: www.ijic._Hlt310507968o_Hlt31507968rg

World Health Organization (2000) *World Health Report: Health Systems—Improving Performance.* WHO, Geneva

World Health Organization (1999*) The Health for All Policy Framework for the WHO European Region*. WHO Euro, Copenhagen

10 Integration: People with autism

Tommy McKay

Autism: the historical development of a concept

In 1943, Leo Kanner, an Austrian child psychiatrist working in America, described 11 children whose socially aloof behaviour and unusual communication patterns represented a new syndrome, which he called 'autism' (Kanner, 1943). Also in 1943, another Austrian doctor, Hans Asperger, lodged a thesis on autism in the University of Vienna, which was published the following year (Asperger, 1944). They had never met, and neither knew of the work of the other. Yet each, at the same time, wrote a seminal paper on an essentially new subject.

While the ideas of Kanner and of Asperger were to have a major impact on future developments in this field, the subsequent fortunes of their respective syndromes were dramatically different. Kanner's autism achieved universal recognition, and served as the basis from which the syndrome was systematically studied and developed in, literally, thousands of studies. On the other hand, when Asperger died in 1980, there was a mere handful of papers recalling his work. It was not until Wing (1981) wrote a clinical account and Frith (1991) provided a full English translation of his work that 'Asperger Syndrome' rose from obscurity to become a major dimension within the autistic spectrum.

Kanner's children were characterised by an extreme detachment from human relationships, failure to use language for the purposes of communication and a desire to maintain sameness, resulting in limited spontaneous activity (Eisenberg and Kanner, 1956). Physical development was normal and

Kanner believed that cognitive potential was good, as seen in islets of normal or superior functioning. While many of his other observations are still central to the current description of autism, it is now recognised that the disorder is associated with significant learning disabilities in up to 75% of cases (Fombonne *et al*, 1997).

The 'autistic spectrum'

Wing and Gould (1979) identified three aspects of development as forming the basis for autism, and it is this triad of impairments in the areas of social functioning, of language and communication, and of thought and behaviour that are now recognised as being both necessary and sufficient for a diagnosis of autism to be made. The clinical picture of the disorder varies considerably from one individual to another, depending on intellectual ability and other factors, and this has led to the concept of 'the autistic continuum' and later of 'the autistic spectrum' (Gillberg, 1991) to express this diversity. At one end of the spectrum are individuals with severe learning disabilities, many of whom are mute (Fombonne, 1999), while at the other are those with Asperger Syndrome, who have no clinically significant cognitive impairments or delays in language development (World Health Organization, 1993; 1992).

Autistic spectrum disorders: an overview

Definition and diagnosis

Autistic spectrum disorders are lifelong, pervasive developmental disorders subsumed under the sub-groups of childhood autism, Asperger Syndrome and atypical autism.

Childhood autism is defined by the presence of anomalous development that is manifest before the age of three years, and by impairments in three areas of functioning: abnormalities in reciprocal social interaction, such as lack of response to other people's emotions; abnormalities in communication, such as idiosyncratic use of language or failure to use gesture;

restricted, repetitive and stereotyped patterns of behaviour, interests and activities, such as compulsive rituals or motor mannerisms involving hand flapping or rocking.

Atypical autism, sometimes described as 'pervasive developmental disorders—not otherwise specified' (PDD-NOS) is the term used when there are factors, such as later age of onset or sub-threshold symptoms.

The nosological status of Asperger Syndrome requires further clarification regarding its essential features (World Health Organization, 1993; 1992; American Psychiatric Association, 1994) and regarding its distinction from 'high functioning autism' (Klin *et al*, 2000). It is characterised by severe impairment in reciprocal social interaction, all-absorbing, circumscribed interests which are imposed upon others in conversation, speech and language problems in spite of superficially excellent expressive language skills, non-verbal communication problems and the likelihood of motor clumsiness (Gillberg and Gillberg, 1989). Unlike autism, there should be no clinically significant delay in cognitive or speech development.

Prevalence

The best current estimates indicate that approximately six in every 1,000 people are likely to have an autistic spectrum disorder. The ratio of males to females is about 4:1 and no social class gradient has been established. The early classic studies, using Kanner's criteria, pointed to a low prevalence of about 4.5 per 10 000 (Lotter, 1967; Rutter, 1966), but the broadened concept of the triad of impairments resulted in a revised figure of 22 per 10 000 (Wing and Gould, 1979). Recognition of Asperger Syndrome added a further 36 per 10 000 (Ehlers and Gillberg, 1993), making a combined total of 58 per 10 000 for ASD. A current controversy in this field is whether prevalence is rising, or if higher reported numbers of individuals being diagnosed are an artefact of better identification processes. Using the figures quoted above, it is estimated that over 300 000 individuals in the UK have ASD, with over 4 million in Europe, 1.4 million in USA, and a world figure of over 35 million.

Causes

ASD is a heterogeneous group of biological disorders for which the causes are poorly understood. Early views implying abnormal parenting as a cause have been abandoned in the light of clear evidence that autism is a neurodevelopmental disorder with a strong genetic component (Medical Research Council, 2001). There is an established link with other disorders, including epilepsy (Wong, 1993), tuberous sclerosis (Smalley, 1998) and Fragile X Syndrome (Bailey *et al*, 1993). There is considerable interest in possible environmental triggers for the disorder, and particular controversy has surrounded the MMR vaccine. However, no association with the vaccine has been established (Madsen *et al*, 2002).

Treatment

A full range of intervention strategies has been used for people with ASD. These include drug treatments, psychotherapy, behaviour therapy and structured educational interventions. Each occupies its own place in an integrated approach to the overall care of individuals on the autistic spectrum. Drug treatments were once used extensively, both in the search for a cure and as a means of controlling difficult behaviour in the absence of more effective methods. These do not offer a long-term treatment modality, but are sometimes an essential adjunct to an overall treatment plan (Campbell, 1989). The earlier widespread, but largely unproductive, use of psychotherapy was based on a model of autism as an emotional disorder arising from adverse early life experiences. However, psychotherapeutic interventions might contribute with specific individuals. People with ASD have an increased vulnerability to common psychological problems, including anxiety and depression, and they require appropriate counselling and support.

In general, the two most useful intervention modes for ASD are behavioural methods and a structured educational curriculum. Behavioural methods are supported by an extensive and enduring corpus of psychological literature covering almost all disorders, and can be a particularly effective support to parents in establishing home management strategies. Nonetheless, structured educational approaches have crucial importance as a treatment modality in their own right. 'Education remains the one treatment approach with the best track record for dealing with the difficulties associated with autism' (Jordan, 1999).

Outcomes

Outcomes for individuals with ASD depend on level of cognitive ability, early development and maintenance of useful speech, severity of original symptoms, and impact of intervention strategies. Those with severe learning disabilities share a similar outcome profile with other non-ASD populations who have equivalent levels of disability in learning; i.e. they are likely to be dependent on high levels of lifelong care and support. Those with Asperger Syndrome, who have higher cognitive functioning, well-developed language skills, and difficulties often not identified before school age, have much more favourable outcomes in terms of independence and access to normal life opportunities. Nevertheless, the common element in terms of outcomes for all individuals with ASD is that their difficulties are lifelong, and even those with more subtle impairments have enduring and often prominent special needs.

It is interesting that, of Kanner's original 11 children who were felt, on the whole, to have indications of 'good cognitive potentialities', only two of those traced 28 years later were in regular employment, while for seven the outcomes were poor, including development of seizures and living in institutional care (Kanner, 1971). A more recent review of more able adults with autism or Asperger Syndrome indicated that just over a quarter were living semi-independently or had paid employment. Only three percent were married, and about a quarter had depression/anxiety or other identified psychological disorders (Howlin, 2000).

Policy, practice and provision

In the UK, as in most countries, there is no autism-specific legislation. People with ASD are, therefore, included in the same statutory framework as others with special needs in relation to legislation on disability, mental health and education. In 1996, the European Parliament endorsed a charter of rights for persons with autism, with a view to its being incorporated within the framework of legislation in each of the member states. The charter embodies many of the principles enshrined in earlier European and UN resolutions on the rights of people with learning and other disabilities, and includes: the right to live independent and full lives; the right to involvement as far as possible in decisions affecting their future; the right to accessible and suitable housing, assistance, equipment and support services and to a sufficient income; the right of equal access to community facilities and services, including transport; the right to meaningful employment and vocational training; and the right to freedom from fear, threat and abusive treatment (European Parliament, 1996).

In addition to the general implications these rights have for society and for public services, there are other specific rights affecting key health and education services. These include: the right to accurate clinical diagnosis and assessment; the right to appropriate counselling and care for physical as well as mental health, and to the provision of appropriate treatment; and the right to accessible and appropriate education.

In promoting these rights, individual countries in Europe and elsewhere have recognised and identified significant gaps in provision for people with ASD, and have responded with local and national policy initiatives. Recognition must be given to the crucial role that has been played in all these initiatives by the voluntary agencies, such as the National Autistic Society, as they have frequently acted as the catalyst for progress, the funders of provision, and the repository of unique and specialist knowledge and skills. Within the UK, national initiatives include good practice guidance on ASD produced jointly by the Department for Education and Skills and the Department of Health (Department for Education and Skills, 2002) and the needs assessment report from the Public Health Institute of Scotland (PHIS, 2001). The good practice guidance focusses on education services as being the key provision for ASD, but emphasises the need for integrated care that involves a multi-agency model of cooperation. This requires a holistic approach to identification, assessment, intervention and support, with key contributions from health, education and social services. The PHIS report identifies current features of service provision and outlines a range of 'ideal' services for people with ASD. The picture emerging, although derived from a Scottish context, is one that is widely reflected elsewhere. In the ASD field, there are substantial gaps at all levels of service provision, across all agencies, all age groups, all categories within the spectrum and all stages of need, from initial diagnosis through to support in adult life.

The range of needs of people with ASD is extensive. While these overlap with the needs encountered by those with general learning disabilities, they call for autism-specific knowledge and interventions to address the triad of social, communication, and behavioural impairments. These impairments have significant implications for the training of individuals and specialist teams to deal with diagnosis, educational placement from preschool through to adult provision, general health issues, family support, including: welfare benefits, respite and residential care and the needs for counselling and therapy. This implies the availability of a very wide range of professionals with specialist knowledge and skills. The list includes: educational and clinical psychologists, specialist teachers, speech and language therapists, paediatricians, psychiatrists, social workers, family support workers, occupational therapists, and specialist nursing personnel.

All major reports highlight ASD as an area in which good protocols have been and are being developed for policy, practice and provision, but major gaps exist at all levels in current services.

Autistic spectrum disorders: the voice of the users

It is inherent within the context of all learning disabilities that the voice of users of services should be heard in relation to any decisions affecting them, but that the very definition of their disabilities represents significant challenges in this area. Often, therefore, it is the voice of representatives and of other affected individuals within families that is heard. Autistic spectrum disorders share many commonalities with other areas of learning disability in this regard, but there are also significant differences. Intrinsic to autism are impairments in insight, understanding and communication, together with a high occurrence of severe disabilities in learning. Opportunities for direct involvement in decisions are often even more difficult for people with ASD than for those with learning disabilities in general. However, the very breadth of the spectrum includes many individuals who are much more able, and who have become vocal representatives and advocates for ASD.

This has become an important feature of developments in the field in recent years and, indeed, is now a significant area within the relevant literature. Authors, who themselves have ASD, in addition to providing informative autobiographical accounts have challenged established views and philosophies, have provided new insights into social and cognitive processes in autism, have contributed to development of policy and provision, and have written advice and guidelines both for professionals and for others with similar disorders (Gerland, 1997; Grandin, 1996; Holliday Willey, 1999; Lawson, 2001; 2000; Williams, 1994; 1992). This includes books written by young people for other children and young people (Hall, 2000; Jackson, 2002).

Autobiographical and other writings by people, who themselves have an autistic spectrum disorder, highlight a paradox in this field of study. On the one hand, they provide a readily accessible means for taking account of the voice of users, and for incorporating their views into service development. On the other, their voices are not representative. They reflect the position and the experience of a very small proportion of the population with ASD, namely, those who are high functioning, who have had the ability to benefit from academic education, who are articulate in their thinking and expression, and who have had both the motivation and the opportunity to turn their views into published works. The vast majority of people on the spectrum are not like this, and much less is known about how their impairments affect them, what their needs are and how they might wish their voice to be heard. Nevertheless, these accounts by users of services have made a distinctive and important contribution to developments in ASD. In particular, they have challenged orthodoxy and have caused many aspects of professional practice and service provision to be re-examined. They have also promoted recognition of the rights and expectations of people with ASD, and the extent to which services and society must adapt to promote their inclusion in the community and to assist them in achieving their full potential.

Current issues and controversies

Autistic spectrum disorders provide major challenges for all who seek to provide a programme of integrated care, whether in health, education, social services, or the voluntary sector. Parents and carers frequently report on the difficulties faced, in particular, at key transition points, such as initial identification of the disorder, finding appropriate educational provision, and then moving on to adult services. Some of these issues are described here in relation to the diagnostic process, the challenge of inclusion, the position of adults with ASD, the philosophy of deviance, training needs and the particular issues faced by those with Asperger syndrome.

Obtaining a diagnosis: the challenge for integrated services

The availability of diagnostic and assessment services for ASD is extremely inadequate and is the source of one of the most commonly reported causes of distress for parents and carers. Despite recognition that autism has a prenatal onset, diagnosis before the age of three years is rare (Baron-Cohen *et al*, 1996), with a reported mean age of around eight years for Asperger Syndrome (Eisenmajer *et al*, 1996). A UK survey of almost 1300 parents by Howlin and Moore (1997) revealed wide regional variations, with many parents experiencing lengthy and frustrating delays and considerable dissatisfaction with various aspects of the diagnostic process, including lack of consistent terminology. The mean age for autism diagnosis was six years but, at the time of survey, the children of many of the parents were already adults, and it was noted that more recent cases were being diagnosed earlier.

While the limitations and potential dangers of labelling people are acknowledged, the importance of diagnosis is central to ASD. It serves many necessary functions, including putting parents in touch with appropriate support networks, pointing to literature that might help to elucidate the disorder, assisting in planning provision, and giving access to particular support services. At times, it is also of direct help to the person with the disorder, providing 'not a label, but a signpost' for understanding the difficulties arising (Jordan, 1999: p30).

The geographical distribution of diagnostic services is so uneven that, in some areas, parents suffer excessive delays, have outcomes in which they lack confidence, and then begin a process of looking elsewhere for further opinions. Often the diagnostician will be the only ASD specialist in an area; for example, a clinical or educational psychologist, a paediatrician or a psychiatrist. Good practice involves a team approach in which there will be a range of professionals from different agencies (Department for Education and Skills, 2002; PHIS, 2001). The lead agent will vary, but is likely to be one of the professionals mentioned, depending on the service that hosts the team. It is necessary, however, that ASD should not be seen as such a specialist area that diagnostic services are few and highly centralised, resulting in months of delay before referrals are taken up. They must become widely embedded within a range of services. This is a key challenge for integrated care and involves organisation of resources and sharing of expertise across services.

Inclusion in school and in society

The concept of education and lifelong learning occupies a central place in integrated care for ASD because:

1) it emphasises the expectation that those with ASD will be in the community and will have the same rights as others to receive educational opportunities;
2) it highlights education as a lifelong process, particularly for those with difficulties in their learning; and
3) educational interventions have the strongest evidence base among ASD treatments.

The foundations for structured educational approaches, as first choice of intervention, were laid in the studies conducted by Bartak and Rutter in the 1970s (Bartak and Rutter, 1973; Rutter and Bartak, 1973). Since that time, the recognition of the primacy of this area has led to a vast expansion of autism-specific educational provision and the transformation of teaching approaches and curricula (Jordan and Powell, 1995). In addition, claims have been made for several specific approaches, including Lovaas, based on applied behaviour analysis (Lovaas, 1987), Daily Life Therapy, using a curriculum delivered through rhythm and movement (Quill *et al*, 1989), and Option, based on adult participation in, and imitation of, the individual child (Kaufman, 1994). While each of these methods incorporates a number of generally accepted principles of intervention, there is insufficient evidence to establish the superiority of any single approach (Jordan and Jones, 1999).

Meanwhile, a worldwide emphasis on social inclusion and participation, as being essential to human dignity and the enjoyment of human rights, has raised the profile of inclusive educational structures. The Salamanca World Statement issued by the United Nations Educational, Scientific and Cultural Organisation (UNESCO) called on governments to 'adopt the principle of inclusive education, enrolling all children in regular schools unless there are compelling reasons for doing otherwise' (UNESCO, 1994: p44). In the UK, this has been reflected in an increasing body of legislation and guidance covering disability and special educational needs. At the same time it is recognised that the spectrum of need, represented by ASD, calls for a spectrum of educational provision. A pattern of provision reflecting increasing levels of need and of the severity of the disorder is shown in *Figure 10.1*.

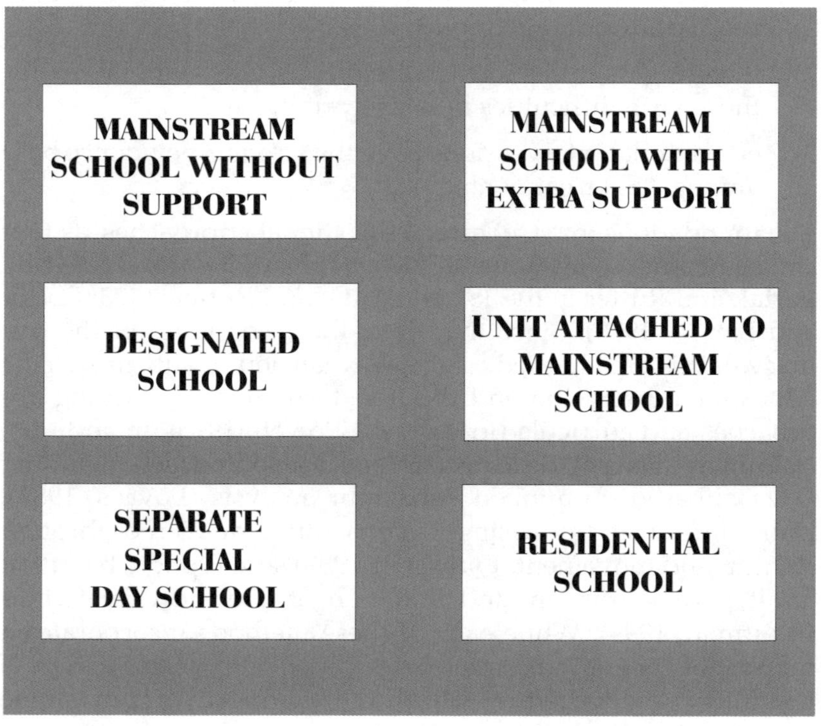

Figure 10.1: A spectrum of educational provision for ASD

Nevertheless, despite the improvements in provision and methods, there are still significant challenges to providing education as part of a framework of integrated care, in ways that will, effectively, promote social inclusion in both school and the wider society. Educational services are over-stretched, autism-specific curricula are patchy, specialist advice and support are unevenly distributed, links between education and other agencies are inadequate, and there is little continuity from school into adult life. In addition, decisions on more extreme forms of segregated provision, such as residential special schooling, are, at times, made because inadequate supports are available locally, while, on the other hand, those who do need a package of residential educational care may not have it because of funding issues across departmental boundaries.

Provision for adults with autistic spectrum disorders

The centrality of education, and the wide expansion of autism-specific educational provision, has led to a major emphasis on children and young people. This emphasis has not been matched in adult provision, with the result that services for adults lag far behind in many key aspects. The relatively recent identification of autistic spectrum disorders began with studies of children, and it is only in recent years that a significant focus has developed on an entire population, which has grown into adulthood with autism and Asperger syndrome. This population requires a full range of services that are often much wider than those required by children, because they include support for independent living, preparation for employment, housing and other issues. It is also a population that, like other people, grows old. There is a crucial need for research to inform understanding and provision for elderly people with ASD.

> *'The principles of care in the community can only truly work if the complex needs of adults with autism are understood and acknowledged'.*
>
> (Peacock, 1996: xix)

Diagnostic services need to be accessible for those whose difficulties have gone either undiagnosed or incorrectly identified through their childhood years. Therapeutic interventions are needed for those who have problems with depression, anxiety and other areas of adjustment, and outreach and support services are required for assisting with the eating, sleeping, behavioural and other problems that occur with a relatively high frequency in the adult population.

Education is also central to the needs of adults with ASD. The association of education with schooling 'has the effect of denying adults with autism access to formal educational opportunities through which their lives could have been enriched' (Jordan and Edwards, 1995: p3). There is a lack of the infrastructure and support needed for successful placement in further education, although models of good practice have been developed (Morgan *et al*, 1996), and there is a general failure to recognise the importance of opportunities for lifelong learning.

The gaps in adult provision at all levels are substantial, and to address them will have considerable resource implications. However, with estimated lifelong care costs for a person with autism and learning disability being almost £3 000 000 (Jarbrink and Knapp, 2001), it is clear that comprehensive, integrated care programmes are not only vital, but are also likely to be cost effective.

'Disordered or different': the philosophy of deviance

Political and professional imperatives in recent years have resulted in more positive viewpoints within society regarding people with disabilities. The move towards social inclusion for all disadvantaged and marginalised groups has raised awareness of their rights and expectations, and has encouraged the celebration of diversity. This, together with the increasing contribution made through autobiographical writings, has had a considerable impact on the study of ASD. The literature of recent years has begun to celebrate the strengths found in autistic thinking, and to promote a view of ASD as different, not disordered. For example, Wendy Lawson, who has Asperger Syndrome, writes:

> *'I do not experience my being autistic as being "disordered" or "impaired" so much as I experience it as being "dis-abled" in a world that doesn't understand autism.'*
>
> (Lawson, 2001: p12)

Lawson has characterised the non-autistic population as being 'neuro-typical' in their development and thinking, and the abbreviation 'NT' has thus gained some currency among both users and professionals. The development of this approach within ASD has both strengths and limitations. As to strengths, as well as respecting the dignity of individuals with ASD, it shifts the focus from a medical model of within-person deficits to an ecological model in which the environment is a key factor. Jordan (1999) has developed the concept of 'prosthetic environments' for people with ASD; i.e. environments that are adapted to support normalisation. For example, within a school or hospital setting, stress may be reduced by allowing an individual with autism to see, in pictorial form, what they are supposed to be doing; where, when, how and for how long.

The limitations of removing the concept of 'disorder' from ASD are also clear. They hinge on the question, 'If it is not a disorder, then why are we trying to fix it?' There is a minority viewpoint among the most able and articulate authors with ASD that autism is one of many differences among people, that it is on an equal footing with other differences, such as race and culture, and that it is, therefore, not something to be 'cured'. However, for most people with ASD, their experience is of the lifelong, pervasive and, indeed, devastating effects of a biological disorder that severely affects every area of their functioning, so that they need high levels of care and support no matter how prosthetic their environment.

The need for multi-professional training

The biggest single challenge to providing integrated care for people with ASD is the need to provide programmes of training across all disciplines. Pre-service training provides only an introduction to ASD within the central professions, such as teaching, psychology, psychiatry, and paediatrics. Most training and experience will, therefore, be developed at in-service level. It is the essential underpinning to diagnosis and assessment, to educational provision, to therapeutic and other interventions, to family support and indeed to all ASD work whether in school, hospital, home or community. Dunlop *et al* (2000) have argued that training should be developed in a context, which is both multi-professional and nationally, as well as locally, coordinated, so that consistent and adequate training programmes may be established.

The special challenges of Asperger syndrome

Asperger syndrome poses a distinctive set of challenges for service provision. By definition, people with this disorder do not have a 'learning disability', since diagnosis requires that they should have no clinically significant cognitive impairment. This has implications for health, social, and education services. The problems incurred by people with autism in their access to health services are often magnified when the diagnosis is Asperger syndrome. The definition of their disorder causes them to fall into the gulf between learning disability services and mental health services. When they do gain access, whether on an in-patient or out-patient basis, they often do not find the skill and specialist knowledge of an ASD team, but are dealt with by services in which there is no clear understanding of their needs and no integrated plan of overall support.

Similar difficulties are encountered in relation to social services. They do not qualify for support from specialist teams dealing with learning disability because of their cognitive level, and, in some cases, the fact that their diagnosis is Asperger's rather than 'autism' denies them access to other supports, benefits, and facilities. Because they are more able, their needs may not be seen as severe enough to qualify for social and family supports, such as respite care and access to befrienders, and yet individuals with Asperger syndrome, and their families, may face long-term, incapacitating circumstances, including severe stress, isolation, and periods of crisis.

Educational provision also provides significant challenges for those with Asperger syndrome. Because of their good ability and language development, they are usually placed in mainstream schools where they are frequently judged by 'normal' rather than 'special' expectations. Their difficulties are viewed as 'subtle' and are, therefore, underestimated. They face higher demands, and their literal thinking and lack of social skills leads teachers to view them as being impertinent or badly behaved. They are motivated to make friends, but lacking in skills to do so. They are also more capable of reflection and aware of failure. For children and young people with Asperger syndrome, school can be a frustrating and isolating experience, accompanied often by difficult behaviour at home and vulnerability to depression and anxiety.

Ideal services for people with ASD

The needs assessment report on autistic spectrum disorders in Scotland set out a number of key principles for the provision of 'ideal' services (PHIS, 2001). It is recognised that, in most countries, the gap between current and ideal service provision is considerable, and that it straddles all care and education agencies. It is also recognised that the move to ideal services raises both resource issues, especially to provide adequate training and to enhance existing provision, and organisational issues, such as reviewing the protocols for interagency collaboration to ensure integrated provision. *Figure 10.2* provides a template for ideal service delivery, and the policies, facilities and resources required to achieve it.

During recent years, there is clear evidence to show that ASD has moved from a peripheral to a central position as a major dimension in the field of special needs (MacKay, 1998). This has resulted in many improvements in service delivery, such as earlier identification and expanded provision, particularly in education services. There remain, however, major challenges to providing seamless delivery of a programme of integrated care in which there is the full participation of service users, their families, the voluntary sector, and the health, education and social services. Autistic spectrum disorders are lifelong and pervasive, but intervention can effect significant change. As one individual with ASD has written, after living for more than 40 years with intense feelings of confusion, frustration, depression and isolation:

> *'This does not have to be the sentence for our children and autistic adults today. With appropriate support and intervention their lives, and those of their families, can be quite different.'*

(Lawson, 2001: p175)

Ideal services should aim to deliver:

- Joint assessment, delivery and review of care in a way that involves the relevant agencies, services and professionals
- Active involvement of the family and, where possible, the individual with ASD
- Early identification
- Appropriate early interventions
- Provision of a range of services delivered seamlessly to meet the various and differing needs of people with ASD, which are planned and developed in a truly multi-agency and seamless way
- Well-planned and sensitive management of the transition between childhood and adulthood within and between agencies
- All planning carried out should place the person at the centre of services and ensure that individual needs are addressed.

In order to do this, services need:

- Joint policies, strategies and operational arrangements between agencies
- An adequate number of skilled and experienced professionals
- Targeted funding for ASD services across organisations, irrespective of co-existing learning disabilities
- A jointly shared record or register of needs of those people currently identified as requiring support because of an autistic spectrum disorder.

Figure 10.2: Ideal services for autistic spectrum disorders (PHIS, 2000)

References

American Psychiatric Association (1994) *Diagnostic and Statistical Manual of Mental Disorders (DSM-IV).* American Psychiatric Association, Washington, DC

Asperger H (1944) Die 'Autistichen Psychopathen' im Kindesalter. *Archiv Psychiatrie Nervenkrank* **117**: 76–136

Bailey A, Bolton P, Butler L *et al* (1993) Prevalence of Fragile X anomaly amongst autistic twins and singletons. *J Child Psychol Psychiatry* **34**: 673–88

Baron-Cohen S, Cox A, Baird G *et al* (1996) Psychological markers in the detection of autism in a large population. *Br J Psychiatry* **168**: 158–63

Bartak L, Rutter M (1973) Special educational treatment of autistic children: a comparative study. I: Design of study and characteristics of units. *J Child Psychol Psychiatry* **14**: 161–79

Campbell M (1989) Pharmacotherapy in autism: an overview. In: Gillberg C, ed. *Diagnosis and Treatment of Autism.* Plenum Press, New York: 203–17

Department for Education and Skills (2002). *Autistic Spectrum Disorders: Good Practice Guidance.* DfES/597/2002. DfES Publications, Nottingham

Dunlop A, Knott F, MacKay T (2000) Can we meet the training needs of professionals working in the field of autism through a multi-disciplinary approach? *Sixth International Congrès Autisme-Europe Book of Abstracts*: 56

Ehlers S, Gillberg C (1993) The epidemiology of Asperger's Syndrome: a total population study. *J Child Psychol Psychiatry* **34** 1327–50

Eisenberg L, Kanner L (1956) Early infantile autism. *Am J Orthopsychiatry* **26**: 556–66

Eisenmajer R, Prior M, Leekam S *et al* (1996) Comparison of clinical symptoms in autism and Asperger's disorder. *J Am Acad Child Adolesc Psychiatry* **35**: 1523–31

European Parliament (1996) *Charter of Rights for Persons with Autism. Written Declarations of the European Parliament, 1996*. European Parliament, Brussels

Fombonne E (1999) The epidemiology of autism: a review. *Psycholog Med* **29**: 769–86

Fombonne E, Du M, Cans C, Grandjean H (1997) Autism and associated medical disorders in a French epidemiological survey. *J Am Acad Child Adolesc Psychiatry* **36**: 1561–9

Frith U, ed (1991) *Autism and Asperger Syndrome*. Cambridge University Press, Cambridge

Gerland G (1997. *A Real Person: Life on the Outside.* Souvenir Press, London

Gillberg C (1991) The Emanuel Miller Memorial Lecture. Autism and autistic-like conditions: sub-classes among disorders of empathy. *J Child Psychol Psychiatry* **33**: 813–42

Gillberg I, Gillberg C (1989) Asperger syndrome—some epidemiological considerations: a research note. *J Child Psychol Psychiatry* **30**: 631–8

Grandin T (1996) *Thinking in Pictures.* Vintage Books, New York

Hall K (2000) *Asperger syndrome, the Universe and Everything.* Jessica Kingsley, London

Holliday Willey L (1999) *Pretending to be Normal.* Jessica Kingsley, London

Howlin P (2000) Outcome in adult life for more able individuals with autism or Asperger syndrome. *Autism* **4**: 63–83

Howlin P, Moore A (1997) Diagnosis in autism: a survey of 1200 patients in the UK. *Autism* **1**: 135–62

Jackson L (2002) *Freaks, Geeks and Asperger syndrome: A User Guide to Adolescence.* Jessica Kingsley, London

Jarbrink K, Knapp M (2001) The economic impact of autism in Britain. *Autism* **5**: 7–22

Jordan R (1999) *Autistic Spectrum Disorders: An Introductory Handbook for Practitioners.* David Fulton, London

Jordan R, Edwards G (1995) *Educational Approaches to Adults with Autism.* Unit 3, Module 1, Distance Education Course in Autism (Adults). University of Birmingham, Birmingham

Jordan R, Jones G (1999) Review of research into educational interventions for children with autism in the UK. *Autism* **3:** 101–10

Jordan R, Powell S (1995) *Understanding and Teaching Children with Autism.* John Wiley and Sons, Chichester

Kanner L (1971) Follow up study of eleven children originally reported in 1943. *J Autism Child Schizophr* **1**: 119–45

Kanner L (1943). Autistic disturbances of affective contact. *Nervous Child* **2**: 217–50

Kaufman B (1994) *Son Rise: The Miracle Continues.* H J Kramer, Tiburon, California

Klin A, Volkmar F, Sparrow S, eds (2000) *Asperger Syndrome.* Guilford Press, New York

Lawson W (2001). *Understanding and Working with the Spectrum of Autism: An Insider's View.* Jessica Kingsley, London

Lawson W (2000) *Life Behind Glass.* Jessica Kingsley, London

Lotter V (1967) *The Prevalence of the Autistic Syndrome in Children.* University of London Press, London

Lovaas I (1987) Behavioural treatment and normal educational and intellectual functioning in young autistic children. *J Consult Clinic Psychol* **55**: 3–9

MacKay T (1998) The education of pupils with autistic continuum difficulties. In: Dunlop A, ed. *Autism: The Way Forward.* University of Strathclyde, Glasgow: 9–23

Madsen K, Hviid A, Vestergaard M *et al* (2002). A population-based study of measles, mumps and rubella vaccination and autism. *N Eng J Med* **347**: 1477–82

Medical Research Council (2001) *Review of Autism Research: Epidemiology and Causes.* Medical Research Council, London

Morgan H, Edwards G, Mason L (1996) Developing a support model, within a further education college, for adults with autism. In: Morgan H, ed. *Adults with Autism: A Guide to Theory and Practice.* Cambridge University Press, Cambridge

Peacock G (1996). Foreword. In: Morgan H, ed. *Adults with Autism: A Guide to Theory and Practice.* Cambridge University Press, Cambridge

PHIS (Public Health Institute of Scotland) (2001) *Autistic Spectrum Disorders: Needs Assessment Report.* Public Health Institute of Scotland, Glasgow

Quill K, Curry S, Larkin A (1989) Daily life therapy: a Japanese model for educating children with autism. *J Autism Develop Disord* **19**: 625–35

Rutter M (1966) Behavioural and cognitive characteristics of a series of psychotic children. In: Wing J, ed. *Early Childhood Autism.* Pergamon Press, London: 51–81

Rutter M, Bartak L (1973) Special educational treatment of autistic children: a comparative study. II: Follow-up findings and implications for services. *J Child Psychol Psychiatry* **14**: 241–70

Smalley S (1998). Autism and tuberous sclerosis. *J Autism Develop Disord* **28**: 407–14

UNESCO (United Nations Educational, Scientific and Cultural Organisation) (1994) *The Salamanca Statement and Framework for Action on Special Needs Education.* UNESCO, Paris

Williams D (1994) *Somebody Somewhere.* Jessica Kingsley, London

Williams D (1992) *Nobody Nowhere.* Jessica Kingsley, London

Wing L (1981) Asperger's syndrome: a clinical account. *Psycholog Med* **11**: 115–30

Wing L, Gould J (1979) Severe impairments of social interaction and associated abnormalities in children: epidemiology and classification. *J Autism Child Schizophr* **9**: 11–29

Wong V (1993) Autism in children with autistic spectrum disorder. *J Child Neurol* **8**: 316–22

World Health Organization (1993) *The ICD-10 Classification of Mental and Behavioural Disorders: Diagnostic Criteria for Research.* World Health Organization, Geneva

World Health Organization (1992). *The ICD-10 Classification of Mental and Behavioural Disorders: Clinical Descriptions and Diagnostic Guidelines.* World Health Organization, Geneva

11 Integrated care for people with mental health and forensic needs

Fergus Douds

This chapter is divided into two distinct sections and will concentrate on the challenges of the integration of people with learning disabilities within society who have some of the most complex needs:

1. Mental health needs;
2. Forensic needs.

Definitions

1. Mental health (psychiatric) disorder: *'Any emotional or behavioural disorder which interferes with, or impairs, the lifestyle and functioning of the affected individual and/or immediate family or carers'* (WHO, 2001)
2. Forensic: *'Belonging to courts of law, origin- held by the Romans in the forum'* (Chambers Dictionary)

1. The challenge of integration for people with mental health needs

Introduction

Why are psychiatrists involved in the care of people with learning disabilities?

In the past, it was thought that people with learning disability did not possess the necessary communication skills to allow full presentation of major mental health disorders. There were also widely held views that people with learning disabilities did not have the emotional capacity to suffer from certain illnesses, in particular, depressive disorder.

People with learning disabilities, however, are not only affected by the same types of psychiatric disorders as anyone in the general population, but, in fact, have higher prevalence rates of some of these disorders. Diagnoses, which would not have been widely considered even ten years ago, are now being made; for example, post traumatic stress disorder, recognising that people with learning disabilities are as prone to psychological/emotional disturbance as anyone in the general population. This does not mean that emotional disturbance should always be assumed as being secondary to a mental health disorder, but it does mean that the presence of such a disorder should be considered.

Under-diagnosis of mental health disorders in people with learning disabilities can often be attributed to a process known as 'diagnostic overshadowing' (Reiss and Syszko, 1983), where possible symptoms of mental illness are attributed to the learning disability *per se*. The only thing that can ever be attributed with certainty to a learning disability is intellectual impairment.

General principles of assessment of mental health problems

The assessment process in individuals with very mild degrees of learning disability will often be similar to that conducted in a general setting, with a focus on a carefully elicited history and attention paid to corroboration obtained from informants. As ability level decreases, particularly with regards to communication skills, the importance of informants, usually family and carers, increases. Obtaining a developmental history is often difficult, due to the passage of time or a lack of familiarity on the part of a carer. It is helpful to try, whenever possible, to obtain information from informants who perhaps have knowledge of the individual in different environments, e.g. at home and at work. If nothing else, this allows one to build up a picture of whether or not behaviours are present in all environments, i.e. are pervasive.

During the assessment, there should be an emphasis on ascertaining whether environmental factors are important, or whether the individual has recently suffered from life events, both of which might help to explain the presentation. Obtaining a good family history is important, given the knowledge that there is a strong genetic component for the major mental health disorders.

The input of a speech and language therapist is especially relevant where communication difficulties are apparent, and an assessment is often helpful to ensure that receptive and expressive language abilities are not over estimated. Multidisciplinary teamwork will always provide the most comprehensive assessment.

Diagnostic interview schedules do exist for use in people with learning disabilities, for example, the Psychiatric Assessment Scale for Adults with Developmental Disability (PAS-ADD) (Moss *et al*, 1993) and, in 2001, a new diagnostic classification system was introduced, the Diagnostic Criteria for Psychiatric Disorders for Use with Adults with Learning Disabilities/Mental Retardation (DC-LD) (The Royal College of Psychiatrists, 2001).

Schizophrenia/other major psychotic disorders

The point prevalence of schizophrenia, among people with learning disabilities, is significantly higher than in the general population, i.e. 2–3% (Lund, 1985; Reid, 1994; Turner, 1989) versus 0.4% (Meltzer *et al*, 1995) and other major psychotic disorders are also over-represented.

It is important, however, to recognise that other mental health disorders are, collectively, more common. In the past, psychotic illnesses have probably been over-diagnosed and antipsychotic medication over-prescribed in people with learning disabilities.

The presentation of schizophrenia and other psychoses in people with mild learning disabilities will often be similar to that seen in the general population, although delusional ideas may be less elaborate and thought disorder less evident. In people with moderate and more severe learning disability, distractibility, covering of ears (due to responding to hallucinations), fear, crying, screaming or talking when no-one is present, social withdrawal and aggression may be seen. In keeping with other mental health disorders, a diagnosis of psychosis becomes more difficult as learning disability becomes more severe. However, it would almost certainly be wrong to assume that people with more severe learning disabilities, lacking communication skills, do not suffer from psychotic illnesses.

Bipolar affective disorder

The lifetime prevalence of bipolar affective disorder in the general population is approximately 1% and it is likely that the rate in people with learning disabilities is at least as high. Diagnosis can, perhaps, be made more reliably than is the case in schizophrenia, by noting the presence of biological features of mania (including increased motor activity, sleep disturbance, disinhibition, increased vocalisation) and depression. In individuals appearing to present with increased motor activity, it is important to differentiate mania from other causes of over activity, e.g. attention deficit hyperactivity disorder.

Depressive disorder

Most studies have found higher point prevalence rates of depressive disorder in people with learning disabilities, than in the general population; 1.3–3.7% (Bouras and Drummond, 1992; Collacott *et al*, 1992; Cooper, 1997; Deb *et al*, 2001; Patel *et al*, 1993) versus 2% (Meltzer *et al*, 1995), an intuitive finding perhaps, given the psychosocial stress and disadvantage that people with learning disabilities often endure throughout life.

Yet depressive disorder is probably under-diagnosed (or misdiagnosed) in clinical practice, due in part to the fact that presentation with some symptoms, such as apathy and social withdrawal, will not always result in acute management problems for carers, leading to no intervention being requested.

As in bipolar affective disorder, diagnosis can be made reliably by noting the presence of biological features, which, in depressive disorder, include loss of interest in normally enjoyed activities (anhedonia), sleep disturbance, loss of appetite, and irritability. Mood often appears more depressed in the mornings and can improve to a degree as the day goes on (diurnal variation). It should be noted that the majority of individuals who suffer from depression once, will have further recurrent episodes.

Care should be taken to differentiate depressive disorder from adjustment disorders. Adjustment disorders are usually responses to adverse life events, e.g. bereavement or acute stress, where there may be a depressive presentation, but this is normally short lived (less than four weeks) and treatment is typically not required.

Anxiety/other neurotic disorders

It should be assumed that people with learning disabilities suffer from the spectrum of neurotic disorders, as they occur in the general population. Neurotic disorders are relatively common in the general population and should, therefore, be considered as diagnoses in people with learning disabilities presenting with emotional/behavioural disturbance. The following prevalence rates were found in a large study of the general UK population (Jenkins *et al*, 1997): generalised anxiety disorder, 3.1%; obsessional compulsive disorder, 1.2%; all phobias, 1.1%; panic disorder 0.8%.

Unfortunately, diagnoses of neurotic disorders depend, to a great extent, on an individual being able to describe his/her thoughts (plus somatic symptoms), thus, as intellectual ability declines, so, too, does diagnostic certainty. Through careful history taking and attentive observation, however, it is possible to consider these diagnoses and provide appropriate treatment.

Dementia *(see Chapter 12)*

In older adults presenting with emotional/behavioural disturbance (or change) for the first time in life, or those with newly diagnosed mental health disorders, dementia should be considered as being a differential diagnosis. Acute confusional states (delirium) should also be considered, given that people with learning disabilities are known to have more physical health problems.

Substance misuse

There has been little published about this subject, which refers to the misuse of alcohol and/or drugs. Substance misuse is endemic in communities, but prevalence in people with learning disabilities is, at present, lower than when compared with the rest of the population (Christian and Poling, 1997). It is possible that this situation may change over time as more young people with learning disabilities receive their education within mainstream schooling, thus exposing them to the range of behaviours experienced by their non learning disabled peers. The possibility of substance misuse should always be taken into account in the assessment and management of mental health disorders.

Autism

People with learning disabilities and autism may present with a range of bizarre, and sometimes bewildering, behaviours. The recognition of autism is, therefore, very important, especially if misdiagnoses of other mental health disorders are to be avoided, notably schizophrenia. It is important to note that individuals with autism may also suffer from any other mental health disorder. Accurate diagnosis of autism and mental health disorders can be difficult; occasionally, empirical trials of medication will be necessary, cautiously implemented and regularly reviewed.

Attention deficit hyperactivity disorder (ADHD)

There has been little research into the prevalence of ADHD among people with learning disabilities (adults). It is necessary to use strict diagnostic criteria, given that over activity and poor concentration are not uncommon features in people with learning disabilities, due to organic brain factors. Even in cases where there is diagnostic uncertainty, it will sometimes be appropriate to instigate treatment for ADHD, although regular review of any prescribed medication will be essential.

Personality disorders

Too often the diagnosis of a personality disorder becomes a pejorative label, which does little to help an individual access treatment or services. In the general population, personality disorder diagnoses have poor inter-rater reliability and in the field of learning disabilities, diagnosis becomes even more fraught and is probably best avoided, except by experienced, qualified professionals.

Other issues

Challenging behaviour

This term is used to describe a wide range of maladaptive behaviours, from minor antisocial behaviours, to serious aggression, including self injurious behaviour. As a rule, it is a term that should only be used when a psychiatric assessment has excluded a mental health disorder.

Behavioural phenotypes

People with certain syndromal diagnoses do sometimes share patterns of behaviour. One of the best examples would be the self-harming behaviour commonly seen in Lesch Nyhan syndrome. There must be awareness of such relationships, but it would be wrong to assume that any described behaviour is a definite part of the phenotype of a syndrome. A carefully elicited history will often help to distinguish between what is phenotype and what is a new behaviour, possibly secondary to a mental health disorder.

Physical health disorders

Consideration should always be given to the state of the physical health of people with learning disabilities who appear to be presenting with a mental health disorder. Physical health problems are often overlooked for similar reasons that lead to mental health problems not being recognised. People with learning disabilities and physical health problems may present only with agitation/distress.

Everyone caring for people with learning disabilities should recognise that, as a group, they are more likely to suffer from poor physical health (Lennox and Beange, 1999). Acute presentation of behavioural/mental health disturbance should always lead to consideration of the presence of medical conditions, particularly illnesses with associated pain. 'Trivial' conditions should not be overlooked, e.g. toothache, dyspepsia and constipation. The potential contribution of sensory impairments should be considered.

Epilepsy

People with learning disabilities have high rates of active epilepsy. Studies have suggested prevalence figures of between 25–35%, compared with 1% for the general population (Coulter, 1993). During the peri-ictal period, individuals may present with a variety of symptoms that could mimic other psychiatric disorders. These include confusion, irritability, aggression, mood disturbance and even psychotic episodes. The potential relationship between seizure activity and behavioural/mental health disturbance must be recognised to ensure that psychiatric misdiagnoses are not made, and that the individual receives appropriate treatment.

General principles of treatment and support

Treatment for people with learning disabilities should be holistic and based on a broader model of care that embraces and takes in to account the biopsychosocial issues.

There has been growing interest in the field of psychotherapies, demonstrating more sophisticated and sympathetic views of mental health disorders and the emotional needs of people with learning disabilities. Therapies, more dependent on communication ability, are used primarily in individuals with mild degrees of learning disability. Art and play therapies, for example, may be of benefit to less able individuals, and behavioural therapies will also assume greater importance for this group.

Social interventions should not be overlooked during treatment. Social isolation, loneliness and boredom are common problems for people with learning disabilities. Thought should be given to the level of support required and to other issues, such as the appropriateness of housing.

When psychotropic medication is prescribed for a mental health disorder, it should be remembered that people with learning disabilities are often more sensitive to the side effects of such drugs. As a general rule, drug dosages should be increased very slowly and the clinician should attempt to maintain an individual on the minimum therapeutic dose.

The individual and carers should be informed about likely side effects, and awareness of the serious extrapyramidal (Parkinsonian) side effects associated with some antipsychotic drugs, which can be irreversible, should be encouraged. There should also be knowledge of the warning symptoms of toxicity associated with other medications, e.g. lithium. People with learning disabilities may need support with compliance and, in some cases, the prescription of liquid/syrup preparations can be helpful. There are psychotropic drugs that require regular blood monitoring and, before their prescription, thought should be given as to whether venepuncture will be possible. As a standard, psychotropic prescriptions should be subject to periodic review by the prescriber.

The importance of the treatment of contributory medical problems, e.g. epilepsy, should be remembered. People with learning disabilities should have the right to specialist treatment and this is particularly important, as a range of health needs can co-exist at the one time.

Developing integrated services to meet the mental health needs of people with learning disability

How will quality integrated services be delivered to the greatest number of people with mental health needs? The answer to this question will take account of the fact that even neighbouring regions may have significantly differing demographics, dissimilar infrastructures and inequities of funding. It is unlikely that rigid adherence to any particular model will result in the provision of an optimal, integrated service.

There should be an emphasis on social integration, productivity, independence and self-esteem. Living in the community and community integration should not be regarded as being the same thing.

A number of principles should apply in order to deliver integrated care, including:

i) *Recognition of the rationale for services to meet the mental health needs of people with learning disability*:

The foundation of any service for people with learning disabilities and mental health needs must first be the recognition that there are high prevalence rates of mental health disorders in this population. If this fact is not taken into consideration, it is likely that service provision will be inadequate. Inevitably, taking account of this fact will have resource implications.

ii) *Community inclusion*:

The locus of care for any truly integrated service will be in the community of the individual with mental health needs, in keeping with the principle of community care. To achieve community inclusion, services need to recognise local differences, including cultural diversity. Knowledge of the community infrastructure is required, in order to develop partnerships that can facilitate community integration.

The fiscal balance of services should be heavily weighted towards community provision, rather than centralised services, e.g. inpatient services. It should not be regarded as generally acceptable practice for individuals to be transferred out of area to receive specialist services.

iii) ***Effective multi-agency working***

The provision of integrated care demands that agencies jointly consider what is best for people with learning disabilities and mental health needs, and work closely together to meet need.

A shift away from the often-artificial dichotomy between what is 'health' and what is 'social' care can only be helpful. A move towards jointly commissioned, resourced and managed services should facilitate effective multi-agency and inter-professional working. Effective joint working should reduce duplication of services and lead to more efficient provision. It should also result in agencies taking collective responsibility for problems. Ultimately, joined-up planning and working by professionals is necessary, if integrated community services are to be provided, drawing on the strengths of professionals from a range of backgrounds.

As well as health and social work professionals, input is also essential from housing and vocational/occupational providers, voluntary agencies, advocacy organisations and other community stakeholders. Appropriate housing and vocational/occupational services are key components of any integrated community service that takes a holistic view of the mental health needs of people with learning disabilities. It is assumed that input from service users, families and carers will be at the centre of all processes.

In practice, effective multi-agency working in delivering often complex packages of care should be cemented by the use of formal operational procedures, e.g. the care programme approach (CPA), (Department of Health, 1990). The CPA highlights multi-agency and interdisciplinary communication; an assessment of the social and health care needs of the individual should be provided and delivered through an agreed written care plan, involving all professional staff, the service user and carers. A key worker is allocated with responsibility for maintaining close contact with the service user, monitoring the delivery of the care plan and taking action, if it is not being implemented. Regular reviews of the service user's care plan and progress should be held.

iv) ***Mainstream versus specialist mental health services***

There has been considerable debate about whether people with learning disabilities with mental health needs should access mainstream (generic) or specialist mental health services.

Some argue that integration can never occur with specialist provision and that such services promote stigmatisation, labelling and negative professional attitudes. Unfortunately, mainstream services have often not responded to the needs of people with learning disabilities. Too frequently, inadequate planning has gone into the provision of mainstream services, which have been difficult for people with learning disabilities to access at a community level. Sometimes, mainstream services have been provided 'by default', i.e. as a result of budgetary constraints. A comprehensive range of services is required to take into account the difficulties faced with assessment/diagnosis and treatment. It is likely that there will be a need for some specialist provision, and people with learning disabilities should have a right to such services. Ideally, mainstream and specialist services should develop and work together by consensus, and seamless cross system access should be a goal.

In the community, there is a need for integrated primary care services to recognise that people with learning disabilities have higher rates of physical illness, and that physical illness impacts on mental health. Ensuring access to a general practitioner is essential, as well as to a range of other health professionals, including, chiropodists, dentists, dieticians, occupational therapists and physiotherapists.

v) ***Provision of lifespan services***

Integrated care is most likely to be delivered by lifespan services. Where age-specific services are provided, clear pathways should exist between services, to limit the stress and inconvenience caused to service users and carers during transition.

vi) ***Support for families and carers***

The provision of integrated community care recognises the value, importance and burden of families/carers, and embraces their needs. Too often, support services for families and carers are provided on an ad hoc basis, if at all. Assessment of the needs of families/carers should be made, such as practical, financial, and emotional support. A range of support services is required, which should include access to respite care where desired.

vi) ***Training, education and research***

Quality services cannot be delivered without adequate attention being paid to the training needs of staff. There should be programmes of continuing training, assessment and professional development for staff. Burn-out and high staff turnover compromise the delivery of quality care.

All services need to be able to demonstrate that care has been delivered appropriately and effectively. Service user and carer feedback should be incorporated into appraisal processes, as far as possible, helping to emphasise that, as consumers, they are at the centre of any service. Outcome data relating to service delivery is increasingly important to satisfy funders and to support development. Services should promote a culture that encourages staff to be involved in research. There is an ongoing need for high calibre research into the mental health needs of people with learning disabilities, continuing to clarify issues, such as prevalence rates, and investigating the differences/similarities between mental health presentations and outcomes in people with learning disabilities, when compared with the general population. Such knowledge should shape service models, helping to improve the quality of care delivered to people with learning disabilities and mental health needs.

2. The challenge of integration for people with forensic needs

Introduction

People with learning disabilities face considerable prejudice and disadvantage, both overt and covert. For those individuals who have forensic needs, this prejudice and disadvantage is multiplied. Surely, there can be no greater challenge than the integration of individuals with forensic needs into our communities.

In the United Kingdom, the closure of the learning disability institutions has, to a large extent, been completed. A significant percentage of individuals living in such hospitals had forensic needs. The closure programme thus marks the beginning of a new chapter in history, presenting society and service providers with fresh challenges. Without innovative and truly integrated models of care for people with learning disabilities and forensic needs, there is a danger that history will be repeated, with insidious re-institutionalisation occurring.

Prevalence of offending

People with learning disabilities are more likely to be victims of crime, rather than perpetrators. People with moderate and severe degrees of learning disability are extremely unlikely to come into contact with criminal justice services.

Research during the twentieth century did appear to suggest that criminal/antisocial behaviour was over represented in people with learning disabilities, supporting the 'wisdom' of previous ages. Such research bolstered the views of eugenecists and was probably reflected in government policies, including the development of institutional care for people with learning disabilities. Over the past decade, these views have been disputed by the publication of studies conducted with greater methodological rigour and through the reappraisal of flawed, or misinterpreted, research. Sadly, many people continue to hold views based on invalidated research findings or prejudice.

There is, however, a growing consensus regarding the prevalence of offending among people with learning disabilities. Firstly, there is broad agreement that the available evidence base cannot support the view that offending is over represented in people that function in the mild learning disability range, and it is agreed that less able individuals are very much less likely to offend. Secondly, it is accepted that people with learning disabilities commit offences across the spectrum of criminal behaviours, except for those offences that require certain skills and opportunities unlikely to be open to people with learning disabilities, e.g. 'white collar crime' (fraud/deception), motoring offences, armed robbery, etc. Thirdly, the evidence for sexual offending and fire-setting being over-represented is weak, although it may be that these offences are over represented in individuals that function in the 'borderline' IQ range; by definition, such individuals are not learning disabled. The definition and ascertainment of learning disability have both been major confounding issues in previously conducted research. Simpson and Hogg (2001) and Holland *et al* (2002) discuss the subject of prevalence in greater detail.

Characteristics of learning disabled offenders

The documented 'characteristics and predisposing factors' in the literature often appear rather arbitrary and are biassed by the geographical context of any study.

Intuitively, one would expect people with learning disabilities, who have offended, to share the characteristics of offenders in the general population and the literature appears to support this. Not surprisingly, individuals will predominantly be young and male, from backgrounds of psychosocial disadvantage, with high incidence of family psychopathology, including offending by other family members. Other consistent findings include: family history of learning disability; poor impulse control; low self-esteem, and behavioural problems dating back to childhood.

General principles of assessment

Assessment is a complex and time-consuming task. The starting point of the exercise may be in respect to the assessment of competence and ability to consent, with regard to criminal justice procedures. Assessment should be seen as being a continuous process. This is especially true of the assessment of risk, which should be evolutionary in nature, constantly informed and shaped by changes of circumstance; for example, responses to treatment.

A thorough assessment process demands multi-agency cooperation and collaboration, particularly with respect to the sharing of information; for example, previous history of offending behaviour and criminal convictions. Assessment should be multi-professional, broad-based and should cover a wide range of factors, including assessment of: psychiatric and physical illness; level of comprehension ability; social/sexual knowledge; skill levels/deficits. Specialist psychological assessment will include a focus on: attitudes, moral development, cognitive distortions, arousal (anger and sexual), and other relevant factors.

Risk assessment

The practice of risk assessment and management is the process of data collection, recording, interpretation, communication and implementation of a risk reduction plan (Maden, 1996). In the field of learning disability, clinical models of risk assessment have become the norm. Instrument-led assessments are not commonly used and, as yet, lack validity in learning disability populations. Any clinical model of risk assessment must standardise and bring together the multidisciplinary collection and recording of data.

General principles of treatment

Can the learning disabled offender be treated? This question may be asked by those who view diversion away from mainstream criminal justice disposals (especially imprisonment) with suspicion, or as a 'soft option'. Of course 'offenders' cannot be viewed as a homogeneous group. Nor, perhaps, is it best that they are always treated in a setting/group context defined by the index offence. Treatment should be tailored to the needs of the individual, encompassing holistic and biopsychosocial approaches.

Appropriate treatment of relevant psychiatric and physical illnesses should occur. As a rule, psychotropic medications should only be prescribed for specific mental health disorders. Antilibidinal drugs are prescribed in some centres for sex offenders, but there is a limited evidence base for their use (Ashman and Duggan, 2002), and increasing ethical concerns about their prescription for people with learning disabilities.

It is likely that treatment programmes will focus on the development of skills, including social, interpersonal, educational and occupational skills. Anger treatment packages should be available given the high rates of aggression among people with learning disabilities seen in a forensic context.

There is a growing literature regarding psychotherapeutical treatment approaches for learning disabled offenders (Beail, 2001; Lindsay *et al*, 1998a; 1998b).

'Treatment' may, at times, have little to do with therapeutic activity and could consist entirely of social interventions, e.g. providing appropriate supported accommodation and structured daytime activity to an individual who has not been in receipt of services, and for whom this deficiency of support was identified as being the most relevant factor in his/her offending behaviour. A thorough multi-agency/disciplinary assessment should identify such needs. It should also flag up other issues that may be very pertinent to the offending behaviour and need focussed treatment, e.g. substance misuse. In the longer term, it is likely that social care interventions will be of vast importance for the majority of offenders, in terms of providing appropriate support and, sometimes, supervision.

Unfortunately, a small percentage of offenders will require secure care for their own safety, or for that of their community. In hospital settings, the level of security and the care plan should both be as unrestrictive as is possible. The unit should be as close as possible to the community of the offender and should

: to maintain a therapeutic milieu, where respect for all individuals is a central tenet of the unit philosophy. Ideally, there should be separate units for young offenders and for women. Advocacy services should be available to all detained individuals.

Developing integrated services to meet the forensic needs of people with learning disability

People with learning disabilities and forensic needs are probably one of the most difficult groups in society to work with. Communities are increasingly intolerant of offenders and taking forward policies of inclusion and integration presents a great challenge to all involved in this field.

A number of principles should apply in order to deliver integrated care, including:

i) ***Community inclusion***

Community inclusion and integration for people with learning disabilities and forensic needs should be a prime goal for those involved in delivering services. A key challenge is how to balance the needs of the individual with the needs of the community. Risk assessment and management strategies need to be combined with care plans that, as far as possible, do not compromise the rights of the individual or the safety of others. Too often offenders are estranged from family and friends and their only meaningful network of support comes from paid carers. The development and delivery of innovative community schemes to support offenders, e.g. 'circles of support' (which are largely reliant on the churches), (Wilson *et al*, 2002), or more secular schemes should be encouraged. Ultimately, any developments that aim to promote inclusion need to grow organically if they are truly dependent on the community, rather than being contrived attempts at social inclusion. Recognising the support needs of family and carers should be central to the promotion of community inclusion.

ii) *Effective multi-agency working*

In addressing the forensic needs of people with learning disabilities, the necessity of effective multi-agency working is, arguably, even greater than is the case in mental health, due to the fact that there are more agencies involved, including the police, prosecutors and probation services. The development of care pathways (for example, Scottish Executive, 2001) is essential to provide integrated and robust care/treatment packages for people with learning disabilities who offend. The entry point of the pathway will often be at the police station, where the presence during the interview of an 'appropriate adult' should be routine for people with learning disabilities, recognising issues of acquiescence and suggestibility.

Jointly commissioned services are, again, most likely to provide efficient and integrated care. Clear lines of communication and information sharing are vital, and organisations must have shared understanding and common goals. Again, the use of the care programme approach (as described in the mental health needs section), or similar procedures, will facilitate effective multi-agency working. Joint working should lead to the development and implementation of common risk assessment and management policies; it should also lead to the establishment of clear pathways between secure and non-secure care, reducing the risk of individuals becoming 'entrapped' in secure units.

iii) *Early interventions*

Service provision should include early intervention packages, targeted towards young people felt to be at high risk of offending, or already in contact with youth justice/social services, as a result of antisocial or criminal behaviour. There is no evidence base to suggest which interventions will have an impact, but it seems likely that many of the treatment approaches currently in use for offenders will be of value. This must be one of the most exciting and challenging areas for professionals interested in this field, and for others in society who want to make a difference. An emphasis on community-based, multi-agency/disciplinary support networks should be a priority. Service provision will need to be robust, flexible and innovative, and it is probable that the professionals employed to deliver an early intervention service will share these characteristics. Any early intervention service needs to be joined up with adult resources, requiring good transition links and processes.

iv) ***Training, education, supervision and research***

The complexity of this client group should demand that only adequately trained members of staff are employed by all agencies, and that there are programmes of ongoing education for all involved in this field. Education should focus on relevant ethical issues. The provision of good supervision is very important, giving staff opportunities to discuss personal issues arising from often difficult work. Team working should be the norm, meaning no one individual feels he or she is solely responsible for the actions of a service user. There remains a great need for quality research into the forensic needs of people with learning disabilities. Long term, multi-centre, follow-up data are particularly required to investigate reoffending, and analyse which treatments/interventions are of most value. To help establish such research, a Forensic Learning Disability Steering Group has been created in the United Kingdom, as part of the National Research and Development Programme on Forensic Mental Health.

References

Ashman L, Duggan L (2002) Interventions for learning disabled sex offenders (Cochrane Review) In: *The Cochrane Library*, Issue 4, 2002, Oxford

Beail N (2001) Recidivism following psychodynamic psychotherapy amongst offenders with intellectual disabilities. *Br J Foren Pract* **3**(1): 33–37

Bouras N, Drummond C (1992) Behavioural and psychiatric disorders of people with mental handicaps living in the community. *J Intellect Disabil Res* **36**(4): 349–57

Christian LA, Poling A (1997) Drug abuse in persons with mental retardation: a review. *Am J Ment Retard* **102**: 126–36

Collacott RA, Cooper S-A, McGrother C (1992) Differential rates of psychiatric disorders in adults with Down's syndrome compared with other mentally handicapped adults. *Br J Psychiatry* **161**: 671–74

Cooper S-A (1997) Psychiatry of elderly compared to younger adults with intellectual disability. *J App Res Intellect Disabil* **10**(4): 303–11

Coulter D (1993) Epilepsy and mental retardation: an overview. *Am J Ment Retard* **98**(Suppl): SI–SII

Deb S, Thomas N, Bright C (2001) Mental disorder in adults who have intellectual disability, 1: Prevalence of functional psychiatric illness among a 16–64 years old community based population. *J Intellect Disabi Res* **45**(6): 495–505

Department of Health (1990) *The Care Programme Approach for People with Mental Illness Referred to Specialist Psychiatric Services*. HMSO, London

Holland T, Clare ICH, Mukhopadhyay T (2002) Prevalence of 'criminal offending' by men and women with intellectual disability and the characteristics of 'offenders': implications for research and service development. *J Intellect Disabil Res* **46**(Suppl): 6–20

Jenkins R, Lewis G, Bebbington P *et al* (1997) The national psychiatric morbidity surveys of Great Britain—initial findings from the household survey. *Psycholog Med* **27**: 775–89

Lennox N, Beange H (1999) Adult Healthcare. In: Lennox N, Diggens J, eds. *Management Guidelines, People with Developmental and Intellectual Disabilities*. Therapeutic Guidelines Limited, Melbourne

Lindsay WR, Neilson CQ, Morrison F, Smith AHW (1998a) The treatment of six men with a learning disability convicted of sex offences with children. *Br J Clin Psychol* **37**: 83–98

Lindsay WR, Olley S, Jack C, Morrison F, Smith AHW (1998b) The treatment of 2 stalkers with intellectual disabilities using a cognitive approach. *J Appl Res Intellect Disabil* **11**: 333–44

Lund J (1985) The prevalence of psychiatric morbidy in mentally retarded adults. *Acta Psychiatr Scand* **72**(6): 563–70

Maden A (1996) Risk assessment in psychiatry. *Br J Hosp Med* **56**: 78–82

Meltzer H, Gill B, Petticrew M, Hinds K (1995) *The Prevalence of Psychiatric Morbidity among Adults Living in Private Households: OPCS Survey of Psychiatric Morbidity in Great Britain*, Report 1. HMSO, London

Moss SC, Patel P, Prosser H *et al* (1993) Psychiatric morbidity in older people with moderate and severe learning disability, 1: Development and reliability of the patient interview (PAS-ADD). *Br J Psychiatry* **163**: 471–80

Patel P, Goldberg D, Moss S (1993) Psychiatric morbidity in older people with moderate and severe learning disability. II: The prevalence study. *Br J Psychiatry* **163**: 481–91

Reid AH (1994) Psychiatry and learning disability. *Br J Psychiatry* **164**: 613–18

Reiss S, Szysko J (1983) Diagnostic overshadowing and professional experience with mentally retarded persons. *Am J Ment Defic* **87**: 396–402

Royal College of Psychiatrists (2001) *DC-LD: Diagnostic Criteria for Psychiatric Disorders for use with Adults with Learning Disabilities/Mental Retardation*. Gaskell Press, London

Scottish Executive (2001) *Services, Care, Support and Accommodation for Mentally Disordered Offenders in Scotland.* Care Pathway Document. Health Department, Edinburgh

Simpson MK, Hogg J (2001) Patterns of offending among people with intellectual disability: a systematic review. Part 1: methodology and prevalence data. *J Intellect Disabil Res* **45**(5): 384–96

Turner TH (1989) Schizophrenia and mental handicap: An historical review, with implications for further research. *Psycholog Med* **19**(2): 301–14

WHO (2001) *World Health Report*. World Health Organization, Geneva

Wilson RJ *et al* (2002) Restorative justice innovations in Canada. *Behav Sci Law* **20**(4): 363–80

12
Integration and older people with learning disabilities

Elita Smiley

Introduction

This chapter focuses on the specific challenges of older adults with learning disabilities and provides detailed information on their physical and mental health needs, as well as the social aspects of ageing. How this relates to service provision and integration is also discussed.

Life expectancy in the developed world has improved considerably and the birth rate has fallen. This has meant that more and more people survive into old age and the proportion of the population of the United Kingdom aged over sixty-five years has risen from five to 15 percent. This change in the age structure of the population and its impact on health and care services has led to an increasing interest in the process of ageing, and its relationship with health. Much of this interest has focussed on the general population. More recently it has also included people with learning disabilities and there is now an evolving body of literature focussing on older people with learning disabilities.

The average age at death for people with learning disabilities residing in hospital has increased from 29 years for males and 36 years for females in the 1950s (Carter and Jancar, 1983) to 66 years for males and 75 years for females in the 1980s (Puri *et al*, 1995). This dramatic change has been partly due to general improvements in health and social care, as has happened for the general population; however, it is also due to a number of factors specific to people with learning disabilities. These include access to medical treatments previously unavailable to them, such as surgery for congenital heart disease, the move from institutionalised living (which potentiated the spread of infection, such as tuberculosis) and the development of more individualised programmes of care facilitating better quality of health care and social fulfilment (Cooper, 1997; 1998). The average person with learning disabilities can now expect to live into middle or old age, which means that the number of older people with learning disabilities is increasing.

It is now recognised that ageing in the general population brings with it a number of changes. These include alterations in personality and attitudes, such as increasing caution, rigidity and disengagement from the outside world, deteriorating physical health, increased risk of dementia and other mental health problems, loss of job, social isolation and increasing likelihood of bereavement. Similarly, most of these changes apply to older people with learning disabilities, which is a very heterogeneous group that also has its own special features. For example, age-related cognitive decline and dementia can affect people with Down's syndrome 30–40 years earlier in life than in the general population. If services are to meet the needs of this population then it is important to acknowledge these differences.

Demographics of older people with learning disabilities

Accurate demographic information on the learning disability population is necessary to assist service planning. However, much of the literature that has attempted to quantify the number of middle-aged and elderly people with learning disability has focussed on differing age groups, or have adopted differing methodologies, making accurate comparisons difficult. Nevertheless, it is clear that there has been a demographic shift in the age structure from a younger to an older population.

A study undertaken by Moss *et al* (1992) looked at the entire population with learning disabilities in the urban district of Oldham in North West England. One hundred and twenty two individuals with learning disabilities over the age of 50 years were identified from the total population of 220 000. The age banding of the whole group was similar to that of the general population. However, the proportion over the age of 70 years was less than that of the general population (due to the higher mortality of people with learning disabilities). Men made up 56.6 % of the group, but the proportion of women increased with increasing age and reflects the increased longevity of women. Most of the individuals identified (75%) were already in contact with learning disability specialist services. This study shows that there are a significant number of older people with learning disabilities and that most are likely to be involved with learning disability services already. Registers or databases of people with learning disabilities have been developed in some areas, with the information used in conjunction with life expectancy and morbidity rates to make accurate predictions for future service requirements.

Mortality, life expectancy and level of functioning of older people with learning disabilities

Although life expectancy for people with learning disabilities has been increasing, it is still reduced compared to the general population (McGuigan *et al*, 1995). Many of the studies looking at mortality rates have focussed on hospital populations and tend to over-represent those who are physically disabled, elderly or behaviourally disturbed. However, recent population-based studies have provided more accurate data and have been large enough to allow classification according to the severity of learning disabilities. Patja *et al* (2000) undertook a nation-wide population study of the life expectancy of people with learning disabilities living in Finland. The mean age of women and men at death was 59.3 and 56 years respectively. The overall mean age of death for people with mild learning disabilities was 58.5 years. The overall mean age of death for people with profound learning disabilities was 46.8 years. This difference in the life expectancy for differing levels of learning disabilities is explained by the physical and neurological disabilities that occur more often with severe levels of learning disability. As a result of this differential mortality, people with more severe levels of learning disability die earlier and the more able and healthier tend to survive into old age (survival of the fittest). This, in combination with continued learning, means that the level of self care skills and competence for the learning disability population as a whole increases with age up to around 60 years. It then tends to decline due to the development of age-related infirmities.

Patja *et al* (2001) investigated cause specific mortality in a nation wide population of 2369 people with learning disabilities. The most common causes of death were cardiovascular diseases, respiratory diseases and cancer. The sample had reduced mortality from cancer and external causes when compared to the general population. Ageing individuals with mild learning disability were found to have similar mortality patterns to the general population. Diseases of the digestive system (such as intestinal obstruction and ulceric perforation) as a primary cause of death were 2.5 times more common than in the general population and associated with profound learning disabilities and being male. Among the elderly, women had an increased risk of fatal fracture compared to the general population. The authors suggested that efforts to reduce avoidable mortality should concentrate on health promotion in the community, reducing accident risks and preventing infections and cardiac diseases.

The physical health of older people with learning disabilities

People with learning disabilities are known to have a high rate of physical disorders. Many will have underlying neurological, hormonal and metabolic conditions associated with the aetiology (cause) of their learning disability. Others suffer from poor health as a result of social disadvantage and difficulty accessing existing health services. As people age, the 'normal' ageing problems of loss of mobility, accidental injury, arthritis, sensory impairment, respiratory problems and incontinence add to this.

As a result of differential mortality rates, it would be reasonable to assume that the physical health of older people with learning disabilities would be better than that of younger people with learning disabilities. However, this does not seem to be the case. Cooper (1998) compared the physical health of 134 adults with learning disabilities living in Leicestershire aged 65 years and over with a randomly selected group of younger adults who had learning disabilities. The older group had higher rates of urinary incontinence, immobility, hearing impairments, arthritis, hypertension, and cerebrovascular disease. Only 17.9% of the older group was free from physical illness compared to 24.7% of the younger group. It seems that the effect of ageing on physical morbidity outweighs the effects of differential mortality. For example, the increased rate of physical illness that comes with ageing has more of an impact on health than the effect of people with more severe levels of learning disability dying at a younger age.

As a group, people with learning disability are often unable to identify or communicate their symptomatology and this seems particularly the case for older people with learning disability. A study by Evenhuis (1997), that looked at the medical aspects of ageing in 70 subjects with learning disabilities over the age of sixty years, revealed that many had marked sensory impairment or quite severe breathlessness, chest pain or urinary problems. However, these subjects had never complained of such symptomatology. They presented more with irritability, inactivity, loss of appetite or sleep problems. Even subjects with mild learning disability and good verbal ability expressed their symptomatology inadequately.

Most people with learning disabilities have to rely on others for the detection of their health problems and subsequent access to appropriate services (Crocker and Yankauer 1987). When successful in accessing health services, their presenting complaints are often different to that of the general population and consequently their symptoms are frequently misdiagnosed or put down to their learning disability (diagnostic overshadowing) and therefore untreated. In addition, studies have shown that, when compared to the general population, people with learning disabilities have a lower rate of uptake of health screening and promotion. These issues become more significant for older people with learning disabilities as the number of health problems they suffer increases with age. Knowing what these health problems are, undertaking regular screening for them and providing education for family carers and health professionals can help to reduce any associated morbidity.

More specific details concerning the common physical health problems that have been identified in older people with learning disabilities are presented below.

Mobility

A higher prevalence of mobility problems is expected in people with learning disabilities as a result of pre-existing neurological conditions or sensory impairment related to the cause of their learning disability, but this increased prevalence increases further with age. Evenhuis (1997) found a prevalence of mobility impairment of 58% in people over 75 years and this is similar to the prevalence found in other ageing populations with learning disabilities. This high rate of mobility impairment, and its potential complications of chronic constipation, osteoporosis, pressure sores, incontinence and deterioration of respiratory function, highlights the need for services to take an active preventative role in this. All people with learning disabilities require regular physical activity and mobilisation, appropriate foot care and walking aids, and adequate treatment of arthritis, osteoporosis and hip fractures. Such a high rate of immobility also has consequences for the design of homes.

Falls and fractures

Among the general elderly population, personal characteristics shown to be related to an increased rate of falls include: age, declining health, being ambulatory, the use of antipsychotic medications and tranquillisers, and female gender. All of these characteristics also pertain to people with learning disabilities, but this group tend to be prescribed more antipsychotic medications and tranquillisers than the general population, which means that they are potentially more at risk of falls. A study by Hsieh *et al* (2001) looked at risk factors for injuries and falls among adults with learning disabilities. It revealed that those who were over 70 years of age, ambulant, and had a higher frequency of seizures were at the greatest risk of injurious falls.

Falls in the elderly can result in fractures. The higher frequency of fractures occurring in females is thought to be due to postmenopausal osteoporosis, which is associated with long-term anticonvulsant use. Because of the increased rate of epilepsy, and thus, also the use of anticonvulsants, people with learning disabilities are at particular risk of suffering fractures as a result of falls. Efforts to reduce the risk of falls and resulting injuries should include optimal seizure control, adequate treatment of osteoporosis, promotion of safe mobilisation and minimisation of environmental risks.

Sensory impairment

People with learning disabilities have a higher prevalence of congenital and childhood hearing and visual impairment. Some as they get older also experience the age-related decline of hearing and vision that occurs in the general population. The available data on the prevalence of hearing and visual problems in older people with learning disabilities suggests that this is higher than for younger people with learning disabilities and slightly higher than for the general ageing population. Certain populations within learning disabilities, such as people with Down's syndrome, are at particular risk of increasing sensory impairment with age. Evenhuis (1995a; 1995b) studied an institutionalised population that was aged over 60 years and found a prevalence of moderate or severe bilateral visual impairment of 27.9% (even with correction glasses) and a prevalence of mild to severe bilateral hearing loss of 33.3% in the age group 60–70 years and 70.4% in those over 70 years. Such high rates of sensory impairment have important consequences on the health and social care of older people with learning disabilities. To facilitate adequate assessment and treatment of such impairments, routine screening of hearing (every five years) and vision (every three years) should be undertaken, with referral to appropriate specialised services when necessary.

Further work on the development of adapted screening methods and screening programmes needs to be undertaken. Older people with learning disabilities should not be excluded from accessing cataract surgery, hearing aids or other such treatments on the grounds of poor co-operation, as with appropriate preparation and support such difficulties can be overcome in most cases.

Incontinence

Several researchers have studied the prevalence of incontinence in people with learning disabilities. Rates increase up to the age of 40 years and then decline before peaking again at 80 years. The second peak occurring at 80 years is similar to that of the general population and is a feature of the increasing infirmity and limited mobility of old age. Cooper (1997) found significantly higher rates of urinary incontinence in people with learning disability aged over 65 years compared to a younger group with learning disability. Evenhuis (1997) found the prevalence of urinary incontinence to be 27% in 70 subjects with learning disability aged over 60 years, and recurrent symptomatic urinary tract infections were diagnosed in 31% of men and 43% of women.

Epilepsy

The prevalence of epilepsy in people with learning disabilities shows a reduction from younger to older groups, again due to differential mortality. There is, however, a peak in the very elderly, which is due to the increased rate of dementia at this age (there is an increased prevalence of seizures in those with dementia). Cooper (1998) found the prevalence of epilepsy in a group of people with learning disabilities over 65 years of age to be 20%, with most monitored by their GP only.

Cardiac and respiratory disease

As in ageing populations without learning disabilities, the prevalence of cardiac and respiratory diseases increases with age. The prevalence rates for older people with learning disabilities are broadly similar to that of the general ageing population, except for hypertension where a reduced rate is found in people with learning disabilities. Evenhuis (1997) found a prevalence of cardio and cerebrovascular disease of 34% in subjects aged 60 years and over, and a prevalence of chronic obstructive pulmonary disease of 16% in females and 35% in males. As found in the general population, chronic obstructive pulmonary disease in this population was related to smoking. Many older people with learning disabilities who are found to suffer from significant ischaemic heart disease or pulmonary disease do not complain of chest pain (even prior to myocardial infarction) or difficulty breathing This illustrates the need for carers to be aware of the risk factors for such illnesses.

Cancer

About half of all cancer occurs in those aged 65 years and over. Common sites for cancer in older people include lung, breast, stomach, colon, prostate and skin. The increased risk of cancer in older people is due to exposure over time to carcinogens and the weakening of the immune system and to hormonal changes that occur with age. These also occur for people with learning disabilities, but the rates of cancer in people with learning disabilities have been shown to be quite different from that of the general population. During a 10-year period, the overall incidence of death due to cancer for an inpatient population of people with learning disabilities was found to be 13.6% of all deaths, compared to 26% in the general population (Cooke, 1997). The ratios of different types of cancer were also very different to those in the general population, with a high proportion being cancers of the gastrointestinal tract. This was also found by Evenhuis (1997). Other types of cancer that are among the most common causes of death in the general population, as detailed earlier, hardly appeared at all in the inpatient population studied. The average age at death from cancer in this study was found to be 62 years for men and 70 years for women.

Breast and cervical screening

Screening is even more important for people with learning disabilities because they have difficulty recognising their own health needs and accessing services. In the UK, all women between the ages of 20 and 64 years, who are registered with a GP, are invited for a smear test every three to five years and all women between the ages of 50 and 64 years, who are registered with a GP, are invited for breast screening every three years. The uptake of screening by people with learning disability is extremely low. Efforts to overcome some of the difficulties include the Good Practice in Breast and Cervical Screening for People with Learning Disabilities document published by the NHS Cancer Screening Programmes. Additional education and awareness for service users and carers is necessary.

Summary

The physical health problems of the elderly with learning disabilities are similar in many ways to that of the general elderly population. They too suffer from the common and chronic health problems of heart disease, respiratory disease, sensory impairment, incontinence and immobility, but probably much more so than the general population. Because of their difficulties in identifying their own health needs and seeking appropriate help, a more proactive role needs to be taken by carers and health services. This should include not only regular health checks and supported access to the same specialist treatments as the general population where appropriate, but also widespread education on the common illnesses that affect older people with learning disabilities and the atypical presentations they may have.

Elita Smiley

The mental health of older people with learning disabilities

Psychiatric disorders other than dementia

The diagnosis of psychiatric disorders in people with learning disabilities can be difficult due to communication problems and atypical presentation of symptoms and history. It is clear from the literature that the rate of psychiatric and behavioural disorders is higher in people with learning disabilities than in the general population. This is due to a variety of biological and social vulnerabilities.

When considering the elderly with learning disabilities, they too have all of these risk factors, but they also have their own additional risk factors that are associated with ageing. These include: increasing physical frailty and pain, sensory impairments, bereavement and loss of previous role, narrowing of social networks and loss of confidence. An increased rate of psychiatric ill health for the elderly without learning disabilities has been demonstrated, but the current literature concerning the elderly with learning disabilities is limited, and differing methodologies, age cut-off points and populations sampled make it difficult to compare studies. However, it is becoming clearer that this population does have significant mental health morbidity and that a large proportion of it is undetected.

In a study of 357 long-stay residents age 40 years and over, Day (1985) found 30% had a significant psychiatric disorder. In a total population survey of 105 people with learning disabilities aged 50 years and over, Moss *et al* (1993) and Patel *et al* (1993) found a prevalence rate of 11.4% for mental illness (mainly depression and anxiety) and 11.4% for dementia. Cooper (1997) examined 134 adults with learning disabilities aged 65 years and over living in Leicestershire and compared this group to a random sample of adults with learning disabilities aged 20–64 years living in the same area. Rates of psychiatric disorder of over 65% (this included 14.9% behaviour disorder, 21.6% dementia) were found in the older age group compared to 43.8% (25.1% behaviour disorder, 2.7% dementia) in the younger age group. The older group had higher rates of dementia, generalised anxiety disorder and a past history of depression when compared to the younger group.

The prevalence of generalised anxiety disorders in people with learning disabilities aged over 65 years is 9% (Cooper 1997). A current diagnosis of depression occurs in about 6% and schizophrenia in 3%. The rates of obsessive-compulsive disorder, mania and autism are similar to that in younger adults with learning disabilities.

Although a progressive decline in behaviour disorders with increasing age has been shown (thought to be due to the physiological changes of ageing making older people less physically active and to the fact that some people gain control of their behaviour as they become older), this was not the case in the study by Cooper (1997). Other studies looking at behaviour disorder in the elderly with learning disabilities have shown that a number of individuals have very longstanding and persistent behaviour problems that have not declined with age.

Detecting mental health problems in the elderly with learning disabilities can be challenging. Any change in a person's behaviour or well-being may indicate a mental health need and requires further investigation. The symptoms of loss of skills, increase or onset of aggression, social withdrawal and poor concentration can be due to number of different psychiatric or physical disorders, and a comprehensive assessment is required to ascertain the correct diagnosis.

Early identification and appropriate treatment of psychiatric disorders can have a considerable impact on the quality of life of older people with learning disabilities. The PAS-ADD checklist (Hester Adrian Research Centre, 1998) is a screening questionnaire, completed by carers, for detecting such problems that has been shown to be of use in this population. Ideally, this should be completed as part of an annual health check for all people with learning disabilities. At times of stress, such as a move of home or death of a parent or carer, individuals should receive extra support to minimise the risk of significant anxiety or depression developing and to ensure early detection and treatment of such difficulties.

Dementia

The issue of dementia in people with learning disabilities has attracted increasing attention in recent years. This has, in part, been due to the association of Down's syndrome with Alzheimer's disease, but it is also a result of the increased life expectancy of people with learning disabilities and, thus, the increasing numbers living into old age and developing dementia, which is closely associated with age. While there has been a large amount of research looking at dementia in people with Down's syndrome, little has been undertaken looking at dementia in people with learning disabilities due to causes other than Down's syndrome.

The estimated prevalence rate for dementia among the general population is 5% in people over 65 years and 20% among those over 80 years of age. The studies of Lund (1985), Moss and Patel (1993) and Cooper (1997), all provide very similar rates for people with learning disabilities when they are age matched, and give a prevalence rate of 22% for those aged 65 years and over. This is clearly much higher than that for the general population and implications for health and social services are readily apparent.

The most common underlying cause of dementia is Alzheimer's disease. It accounts for approximately 50% of dementias. Down's syndrome is known to be associated with Alzheimer's disease. Almost all people with Down's syndrome over the age of 40 years have neuropathological changes similar to those seen in Alzheimer's disease. However, not all have the clinical features of dementia and, indeed, some people with Down's syndrome survive into their 50s and 60s without developing dementia. Age specific rates for dementia in people with Down's syndrome increase from 1–2% at 30–40 years to 40% at 50–60 years (Holland *et al*, 1998). The average age of onset for clinical manifestations of Alzheimer's disease in individuals with Down's syndrome is between 51 and 54 years. The age of onset of dementia for individuals with learning disabilities as a result of other causes tends to be over 65 years.

Dementia is defined as a syndrome due to disease of the brain, usually of a chronic or progressive nature, in which there is disturbance of multiple higher cortical functions, including memory, thinking, orientation, comprehension, calculation, learning capacity, language, and judgement. A clinical diagnosis of dementia in the non-learning disabled population is based on the evidence of progressive deterioration in cognitive abilities and daily living skills. In people with learning disability, the pre-morbid cognitive functioning and daily living skills are often at a different level, thus identifying changes in this way is not helpful. Clinicians are required to look more for a change from a person's baseline level of functioning. If there is no previous documented level of functioning, this can be difficult and sometimes leads to delayed diagnosis and treatment. It has been recommended that all people with learning disabilities be evaluated at least once in early adulthood (by age 25 years), using standardised psychological procedures to establish a record of baseline functioning, which would then serve as each individual's own point of reference when a diagnosis of dementia is being considered (Alwyrd *et al*, 1997). This has significant resource implications. However, in the long term it would improve the detection, diagnosis and treatment of dementia in people with learning disabilities. A working group for the establishment of criteria for the diagnosis of dementia in individuals with learning disability, set up under the auspices of the International Association for the Scientific Study of Intellectual Disability [IASSID] group (Alwyrd *et al*, 1997), has published standardised criteria for the diagnosis of dementia in people with learning disabilities. It is intended that the development of the new diagnostic criteria will facilitate communication among researchers and clinicians, thereby leading to further progress in the knowledge of dementia in people with learning disabilities.

Recognising dementia in people with learning disabilities

It has been suggested that the clinical presentation of dementia among adults with learning disabilities, at most levels of learning disabilities, is similar to that of adults without learning disabilities (Janicki and Dalton, 1999). The first noticeable change that occurs is often in memory; for example, the inability to remember social arrangements, the location of recently placed objects, or the day's events. This increases the need for prompting to remember the steps required to perform previously acquired tasks, with the failure to recognise friends and family indicating more severe memory loss. Changes in mood and emotional impulse control become apparent as the dementia progresses, as well as in motivation and general interest. Disorientation for time and place may occur and, as a result, wandering can be problematic. As the dementia progresses further, skills with language are lost and the person experiences feeding difficulties and gait deterioration. As the terminal stage of the illness approaches, urinary incontinence and the loss of most motor functions necessitates total nursing care. Frequently there is a general increase in muscle tone and myoclonic jerks or generalised seizures may occur (particularly in people with Down's syndrome). The average duration of the illness is ten years, with the need for quality nursing care as the disease progresses, when there is complete physical dependency. Psychotic symptoms, such as persecutory delusions and auditory and visual hallucinations, or significant depressive and anxiety symptoms occur in many cases and can lead to difficult behaviour. The diagnosis of dementia cannot be made until other illnesses that mimic dementia, such as depression or hypothyroidism, have been excluded. This necessitates an extensive assessment, including a number of investigations.

Treatment

The approach to the treatment and support of people with learning disability and dementia should be multidisciplinary, and include a variety of treatment methods and options. Education and carer support, including contact with voluntary organisations, such as the Alzheimer's Disease Society and regular respite care, are particularly important. Sufferers should continue with recreational and occupational activities for as long as possible and early arrangements should be made to cope with their increasing support needs.

Drugs for the treatment of the cognitive symptoms in Alzheimer's disease are now available. However, their use in treating people with learning disabilities has not as yet been fully evaluated. Provisional results suggest that they may be of some use.

Services

At present, it is old age psychiatry services that have most experience and expertise in dealing with dementia. However, the majority do not provide services for elderly people with learning disabilities or for people with dementia aged less than 65 years. In the United Kingdom, the majority of older people with learning disabilities receive their psychiatric care and treatment for dementia through specialist learning disability services (Bailey and Cooper, 1997; Smiley *et al*, 2002). These services are predominantly provided separately from mainstream old age psychiatric services. Due to the limited numbers of cases and lack of experience and resources of many learning disability services in treating dementia, this may not be the best arrangement. The fact that the course of dementia in people with learning disabilities is similar to that of the general population supports the use of mainstream services as opposed to specialist services. However, there are some concerns that inexperienced staff in old-age services will inadvertently attribute health needs of people with learning disabilities to their learning disability. Models of care that enable close collaboration between both old age and learning disability services, with the sharing of information and resources where appropriate, is suggested as the best way forward for the management of dementia in people with learning disabilities, but further research into this topic is required.

Social aspects of ageing

In addition to cognitive decline and an increased risk of physical and mental health problems, ageing brings with it a number of social and economical changes, the most obvious being that of retirement. Retirement is a welcome event for many people, providing the opportunity for indulgence in leisure activities previously hampered by the demands and structure of work. However, for people with learning disabilities, the transition is often non-existent, confusing or frightening and for many a job has never been a reality and 'work' has often meant activities undertaken at day centres. People with learning disabilities have often, in the past, had no formal paid work to retire from, or they are not allowed to retire with continued attendance at a day centre being a condition of their care package.

Ashman *et al* (1995) investigated the employment and retirement status of people with learning disabilities aged over 55 years living in two Australian states. A large number of the participants had never been involved in full- or part-time employment. Those that were in work expressed concern about the prospect of retirement and the loss of income associated with this. Recent changes in policy and increasing programmes of supported employment for people with learning disabilities will result in the next cohort of elderly people with learning disabilities being much more likely to have employment to retire from and the need for pre-retirement programmes will increase.

As with other retirees, older people with learning disabilities are faced with the challenge of finding meaningful and enjoyable activities to fill their leisure time. It is recognised that higher levels of leisure participation are associated with higher perceived life satisfaction among older adults with learning disabilities. A qualitative study on the nature of leisure activities of older adults with learning disabilities (Rogers *et al*, 1998) revealed that care providers decided the nature of their leisure activities for all participants. The majority of participants desired greater freedom and control of their leisure activities. Only a few of the participants were satisfied with life in retirement. For those who were satisfied, continued or increased involvement in community activities was the key element. It is thus important that older people with learning disability have continued opportunities for varied and fulfilling leisure activities. Services must take this into consideration when developing care packages and community support needs.

As people age, so do their friends and family and this brings an increasing risk of bereavement and loss. For many adults with learning disabilities, loss of a parent also results in loss of residence and a change in carer (Hollins, 1997). The combined effect of this increases their vulnerability and consequently many will develop significant emotional and behavioural problems following bereavement. For many, exclusion from the normal grieving process and attendance at the funeral further hampers their difficulties in adjusting to the death of a loved one. Carers and health professionals should be alert to the potential bereavements their clients may suffer and attempt to minimise the impact of this by facilitating adequate preparation and involvement in the process where possible. Another difficulty that often follows the death of a family member is the loss of information with that person, such as a person's likes and dislikes, best means of communication and life events, etc. Keeping a life storybook is one way of avoiding this. There are now several published resources that can help support people with learning disabilities, and this includes the successful series, 'Books Beyond Words' by Sheila Hollins and colleagues, jointly published by St George's Hospital Medical School and the Royal College of Psychiatrists.

Meeting the health needs of older people with learning disability

While it is accepted that older people with learning disabilities have higher rates of physical and mental health problems than younger people with learning disabilities, and that many of these problems are undetected and untreated, how best to meet these needs and provide support is less clear. Although older people with learning disabilities suffer from similar health problems to older people without learning disabilities, the particular vulnerabilities and atypical presentations that occur in people with learning disabilities often results in them receiving poor or inadequate health care when it is provided by professionals unaware of these special features. Specialised services can reduce this risk and deliver appropriate care. However, the issues of inclusion must be addressed.

There is increasing research in the United States on the needs of older people with learning disabilities. Janicki *et al* (1995) advocated the integration of services for reasons of non-discrimination and funding. They found some success with this, but Seltzer (1988) had different findings. He looked at the service use of all people, aged 55 years and over, with learning disabilities, who received services in Massachusetts. He used a telephone survey to assess age-integrated (learning disability service providing for all ages), age specialised (learning disability service for the elderly) and generic (services for the general elderly population) services. The results indicated that the most prominent weakness of age-integrated services was that they did not provide age-appropriate activities. The activities were too pressurised and insufficiently sensitive to clients' health needs. Although the generic ageing services offered age-appropriate programs, these were not suitable for individuals with learning disabilities as they were focussed at an inappropriate cognitive level or were in large groups. There were also concerns at the lack of expertise in supporting people with learning disabilities. Age-specialised services had the greatest number of strengths identified. Retirement options were more likely to be offered to clients and the services were more likely to have expertise in both aging and learning disabilities.

Although age specialised services may be the ideal, for many rural areas and services with limited resources, small numbers of older people with learning disabilities can make such services unrealistic and unlikely. The Department of Health (2001) highlights the importance of mainstreaming where this is appropriate. The Scottish Executive (2000) stresses the importance of working in partnership, with access to specialist learning disabilities health services when indicated on the basis of individual need. How services interpret and respond to such policies will depend more on their own local resources, practices and local policies. Some services in the UK are developing plans to create special services for older people with learning disabilities, but whether this becomes a reality and provides better care for these people will require the passage of time and further research to decide.

Conclusions

Meeting the health and social needs of the increasing number of older people with learning disabilities poses new and considerable challenges. Clearly some have significant physical and mental health needs that are similar to those of the general ageing population. However, it is also important to recognise that some have special needs that, at times, makes accessing mainstream services inappropriate. In addition to deteriorating health, older people are faced with reduced leisure opportunities, social isolation, an increased risk of bereavement and/or having to move home. Carers and health professionals working with older people with learning disabilities need to take account of these complex issues when planning health and social care services for older people with learning disabilities. Regular health screening and attention to preventative measures are necessary. Forming and maintaining close links with mainstream services, including supported access where appropriate, is vital to ensure that older people with learning disabilities receive the same quality of health care as older people in general. Simply being aware of how ageing effects people with learning disabilities, and the common health and social problems from which they suffer, is the first step in providing comprehensive health care in whatever setting. Education and awareness of the needs of older people with learning disabilities are the key issues.

References

Alwyrd E, Burt D, Thorpe L *et al* (1997) Diagnosis of dementia in individuals with intellectual disability: report of the task force for development of criteria for diagnosis of dementia in individuals with mental retardation. *J Intellect Disabil Res* **41**: 152–64

Ashman AF, Suttie JN, Bramley J (1995) Employment, retirement and elderly persons with an intellectual disability. *J Intellect Disabil Res* **39**: 107–15

Bailey N, Cooper S-A (1997) The current provision of specialist health services to people with learning disabilities in England and Wales. *J Intellect Disabil Res* **41**: 52–59

Carter G, Jancar J (1983) Mortality in the mentally handicapped: a fifty year survey of the Stoke Park Group Hospitals (1930–1980). *J Ment Defic Res* **27**: 142–56

Cooke LB (1997) Cancer and learning disability. *J Intellect Disabil Res* **41**: 312–16

Cooper SA (1998) Clinical study of the effects of age on the physical health of adults with mental retardation. *Am J Ment Retard* **102**: 582–89

Cooper SA (1997) Epidemiology of psychiatric disorders in elderly compared with younger adults with learning disabilities. *Br J Psychiatry* **170**: 375–80

Crocker AC, Yankauer A (1987) Basic issues. *Ment Retard* **25**: 227–32

Day K (1985) Psychiatric disorder in the middle-aged and elderly mentally handicapped. *Br J Psychiatry* **147**: 660–67

Department of Health (2001) *Valuing People: A New Strategy for Learning Disabilities.* HMSO, London

Evenhuis HM (1997) Medical aspects of ageing in a population with intellectual disability: III. Mobility, internal conditions and cancer. *J Intellect Disabil Res* **41**: 8–18

Evenhuis HM (1995a) Medical aspects of ageing in a population with intellectual disability: I Visual impairment. *J Intellect Disabil Res* **39**: 19–25

Evenhuis HM (1995b) Medical aspects of ageing in a population with intellectual disability: II Hearing impairment. *J Intellect Disabil Res* **39**: 27–33

Hester Adrian Research Centre (1998) *The PAS-ADD Checklist*, University of Manchester, Manchester

Holland AJ, Hon J, Huppert FA *et al* (1998) Population-based study of the prevalence and presentation of dementia in adults with Down's syndrome. *Br J Psychiatry* **172**: 493–98

Hollins S, Esterhuyzen A (1997) Bereavement and grief in adults with learning disabilities. *Br J Psychiatry* **170**: 497–501

Hsieh K, Heller T, Miller AB (2001) Risk factors for falls among adults with developmental disabilities. *J Intellect Disabil Res* **45**: 76–82

Janicki MP, Ackerman L, Jacobson W (1985) State developmental disabilities/ageing plans and planning for an older developmentally disabled population. *Ment Retard* **23**: 297–301

Janicki MP, Dalton AJ (1999) Dementia in developmental disabilities. In: Bouras N, ed. *Psychiatric and Behavioural Disorders in Developmental Disabilities and Mental Retardation*. Cambridge University Press, Cambridge: 121–53

Janicki M, Heller T, Seltzer G *et al* (1995) *Practice Guidelines for the Clinical Assessment and Care Management of Alzheimer and other Dementias among Adults with Mental Retardation*. American Association on Mental Retardation, Washington DC

Lund J (1985) The prevalence of psychiatric morbidity in mentally retarded adults. *Acta Psychiatr Scand* **72**: 563–70

McGuigan SM, Hollins S, Attard M (1995) Age specific standardized mortality rates in people with learning disability. *J Intellect Disabil Res* **39**: 527–31

Moss S, Goldberg D, Patel P, Wilkin D (1993) Physical morbidity in older people with moderate, severe and profound mental handicap, and its relation to psychiatric morbidity. *Social Psychiatry Psychiatr Epidem* **28**(1): 32–39

Moss S, Patel P (1993) The prevalence of mental illness in people with intellectual disability over 50 years of age, and the diagnostic importance of information from carers. *Ir J Psychol Med* **14**: 110–29

Moss S, Hogg J, Horne M (1992). Demographic characteristics of a population of people with moderate, severe and profound intellectual disability (mental handicap) over 50 years of age: age structure, IQ and adaptive skills. *J Intellect Disabil Res* **36**: 387–401

Patel D, Goldberg D, Moss S (1993) Psychiatric morbidity in older people with moderate and severe learning disability. II: The prevalence study. *Br J Psychiatry* **163**: 481–91

Patja K, Iivanainen M, Vesala H *et al* (2000) Life expectancy of people with intellectual disability: a 35-year follow-up study. *J Intellect Disabil Res* **44**: 591–99

Patja K, Molsa P, Iivanainen M (2001) Cause specific mortality of people with intellectual disability in a population-based, 35 year follow-up study. *J Intellect Disabil Res* **45**: 30–40

Puri BK, Lekh SK, Langa A, Zaman R, Singh I (1995) Mortality in a hospitalized mentally handicapped population:a 10 year survey. *J Intellect Disabil Res* **39**: 442–46

Rogers NB, Hawkins BA, Eklund SJ (1998) The nature of leisure in the lives of older adults with intellectual disability. *J Intellect Disabil Res* **42**: 122–30

Scottish Executive (2000) *The Same as You? A Review of Services for People with Learning Disabilities.* The Stationary Office, Edinburgh

Seltzer M (1988) Structure and patterns of service utilization by elderly persons with mental retardation. *Ment Retard* **26**: 181–85

Smiley E, Cooper S-A, Miller SM *et al* (2002) Specialist health services for people with intellectual disability in Scotland. *J Intellect Disabil Res* **46**: 1–9

Glossary of terms

Advocate	A person who helps others make decisions about their lives and have their say about what they want to happen in their lives
Asperger's syndrome	A form of Autism that affects people of average or above average intelligence
Autism	A lifelong developmental disability that impacts upon the way a person communicates and relates to others. Not all people with Autism have a learning disability
Autosomes	The chromosomes other than the sex chromosome. Each member of an autosome pair (in diploid organisms) is of similar length and in the genes it carries
Care Programme Approach (CPA)	An approach to managing the care of people with the most complex needs to ensure an assessment of need and care plan are in place and reviewed at predetermined times
Challenging behaviour	A term used to describe when a person is acting in such a way that might cause harm to him/herself or to others
Cloning	The transference of a DNA sequence from one organism to another that has been replicated by genetic engineering techniques
Cognitive	The process of knowing and understanding that includes aspects, such as awareness, perception, reasoning, and judgment
Community care	The assessment of need and commissioning of packages of care to support people to live as independently as possible within their community
Complex needs	The term used to describe people who have additional needs beyond their learning disability

Dementia	A condition that is characterised by deterioration in memory, social functioning and the ability to self care and make independent decisions overtime. Some people with learning disabilities can suffer from early onset dementia, for example those with Down's syndrome
Diagnostic overshadowing	The term used to describe the inability to see ill-health and conditions that may be present in a person beyond the learning disability
Differential diagnosis	The range of possible diagnostic options available within a range of conditions and diseases.
Discrimination	The ability and power to make distinctions about the treatment of and value of particular groups of people or individuals within society
Disorder	A deviation from a person's normal physical or mental health
DNA	Deoxyribonucleic acid—A nucleic acid that carries the genetic information in the cell and is capable of self-replication and synthesis of the RNA
Dual diagnosis	The term used to describe a person who has a learning disability and mental health problems
Forensic	The assessment, diagnosis and treatment of a person who has a mental disorder and is also charged with or has been convicted of a criminal offence
Genetics	The biological characteristics inherited by an individual
Health check	A form of assessment that seeks to identify unrecognised and unmet health needs
Health promotion	Structured activities aimed at improving overall health and well being
Integration	The inclusion of people of minority groups into unrestricted and equal membership of society

Learning disability	A significant lifelong condition that is present on or around the time of birth and before adulthood and affects development, the ability to understand information, learn skills and cope independently
Mainstream	Services that are available to all members of the community
Mental health	A person's overall emotional and psychological condition
Mutation	A change in the DNA sequence within a chromosome of an organism that results in the creation of a new character or trait not found in the parent
Offending behaviour	The term used to describe actions that are against criminal law
Phenylketonuria	A genetic disorder in which the body lacks the enzyme necessary to metabolise the substance phenylalanine to tyrosine. If not treated, brain damage and progressive learning disability result, due to the accumulation of phenylalanine and its breakdown products
Policy	A plan or course of action, of a government, political party, or business organisation that is intended to influence the decisions and actions of others
Profound and multiple impairment	A person with a severe learning disability that is characterised by a range of complex needs that can include physical and sensory impairment
Psychotherapy	A form of psychological treatment used to help people understand what has been happening in their lives and look at ways to make changes
RNA	Ribonucleic acid—A long, single-stranded chain of alternating phosphate and ribose units with the bases adenine, guanine, cytosine, and uracil bonded to the ribose
Sensory impairment	A loss of sight or hearing or both

Social inclusion	Where all people can live in and be part of the community, free from discrimination and injustice
Syndrome	A group of symptoms and characteristics that result in a specific condition. The most common syndrome being Down's syndrome.
Therapeutic interventions	A range of treatment that includes drugs, physical and psychological therapy aimed at improving health and well-being

Index